THE HEALING POWER WITHIN

TRANSFORMING CANCER TO WELLNESS

Shruti SETHI

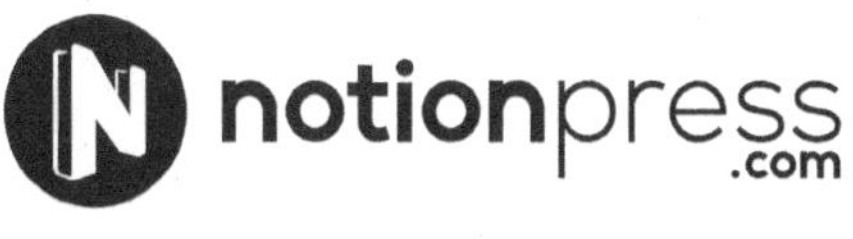

INDIA · SINGAPORE · MALAYSIA

ISBN 979-8-89277-796-4

Contents

Chapter 1
A Bomb Dropped

April 17, 2016

To be 34, with a successful career in fashion in Mumbai, married and well-settled, with good friends, and in the prime of health—this was supposed to be the definition of living my best life. However, life has a knack of defying my grand plans. Though some small aspects had gone askew, so far they hadn't shaken my resolve. Little did I suspect that a grand upheaval was just around the corner, waiting to turn my world entirely on its head!

By the time I was 27, my dream of marriage had become a reality, but parenthood remained elusive. Five years into a marriage I had chosen, my once-promising world began unravelling at the seams. The initial years of matrimony proved tumultuous, marked by fights and arguments that went beyond the usual relationship strife. I could tolerate the disagreements but I could no longer endure the physical assault. I made every effort to mend the fractures in our marriage and forgave my husband repeatedly, but eventually a tipping point arrived. Soon, the toxicity of the relationship became too much to handle. The marriage was sapping my happiness and draining my vitality, forcing me to look for a way out.

I separated from my husband and moved in with my aunt, in keeping with the legal requirement of a reasonable separation period before initiating divorce proceedings. I was determined to craft a new chapter in my life, and I embarked on a journey towards independence, settling into a cosy condo in Bandra. Armed with new possessions, I saw this as a fresh beginning. Simultaneously, I took up work as a fashion consultant with a start-up to bolster my income. However, the internal politics there proved too stressful, prompting me to resign within three months.

Reflecting on my journey, I realize I have consistently chosen the more challenging path, be it in matters of the heart, professional pursuits, or in other facets of life. Yet, I found adapting to this new phase most challenging. Solo living was a significant transition, and I was struggling to acclimatize. Just as I was settling into this unfamiliar territory, life delivered a staggering blow—CANCER. It crept into my body like a secret invader. I couldn't figure out how long it had been silently devouring my cells. I had many plans for my life, but it seemed God had decided to present me with a formidable test. Little did I realize then that my relationship status was not the only thing about to go through the blender!

So, how did I discover the truth? I regarded myself as healthy, having never grappled with any significant medical issues. I was neither overweight nor had I ever indulged in smoking or drinking a lot. Physical activity was a part of my routine—regular Zumba classes, yoga sessions, and badminton. Yet, over the past year, my body had been sending me distress signals. I felt unwell often; a rash appeared on my skin, and the skin on my hands and feet began to flake causing excruciating pain. Bloating became an unwelcome companion, and my Vitamin D3 levels dropped to a new low.

One day, my fingers discovered an unfamiliar presence on the right side of my neck—a conspicuous pinkish-red lump. Initially, I dismissed it as the aftermath of a strenuous badminton game, attributing it to awkward neck motion. But, over the following days, I battled a fatigue that forced me to summon every ounce of strength to rise from my bed, only to remain sleepless at night. Determined to defy the looming lethargy, I maintained physical activity, although concentration became increasingly difficult.

My mother flew down from the United States for a family wedding in the first week of March. The week leading up to the wedding was when the mysterious lump appeared. I chose to ignore the lump and savour the festivities instead. However, as the wedding unfolded, the unrelenting fatigue began to take its toll. Dancing was an activity I had always enjoyed, but rehearsals for the Sangeet ceremony felt gruelling. At night, sleep eluded me, and facing relatives who were privy to my divorce proceedings posed an additional challenge. Although no one commented, attending a wedding as a solo entity after always appearing on these occasions as a couple with my ex, felt surreal. Amidst these emotions, an uncharacteristic craving for sweets took hold, a departure from my customary restraint. I wondered whether this was a manifestation of emotional eating or my body's plea for solace in sugar.

Meanwhile, I was in the midst of shifting houses, craving a space to call my own. I rented a studio apartment where clients could readily visit as I transitioned into crafting exquisite attire and bridalwear from home.

Seeking relief from my symptoms, I experimented with various remedies—from balms and sprays to the contrasting sensations of hot and cold water therapy. The lump proved stubborn; its ominous presence persisted, dashing my hopes for a swift resolution. Even alternative therapies like acupuncture and Sujok provided no respite. I could no longer sleep on my right side. In desperation, I reached out to a trusted physician friend who urged me to get an X-ray. Reluctantly, I complied. As the X-ray technician scrutinized the images, he noted something unsettling—a discernible movement or indication of an unseen intruder, possibly tuberculosis.

Following an examination, my physician friend recommended Fine Needle Aspiration Cytology (FNAC), a procedure to sample superficial masses, like the one in my neck. Typically conducted at outpatient clinics, FNAC causes patients minimal discomfort and has a virtually zero risk of complications. I agreed to the proceeding. What followed was a painful ordeal! A formidable, needle-like instrument pierced the lump, extracting vital liquid. My cries echoed through the room, and were so overwhelming that my sister, who had accompanied me, nearly fainted.

A week later, the results were ready. I went to NM Medical in Bandra to collect them, confident that they would report some trivial concern. However, as I read the report, shockwaves went through me—it suggested the possibility of Hodgkin's Lymphoma. I surrendered to my habit of turning to Google. The word 'CANCER' ensnared my thoughts, echoing incessantly in my mind. I must have scrutinized it a hundred times, an avalanche of emotions pouring over me. I did not know how to react or what steps to take. I was taking acupressure and acupuncture treatments to counter my fatigue, so I made my way there in a daze. Around five in the evening, I dialled my parents in New York to deliver the devastating news. As the conversation unfolded, my vision blurred, and saltiness filled my mouth as my tears flowed freely. My parents were shattered by the revelation but tried to cloak their anxiety beneath a veil of reassurance.

I convinced myself this had to be a dreadful dream, and I would awaken to find everything miraculously restored to normal. But that wasn't to be. I shared the report with my physician and he urged me towards a biopsy—a procedure that involves the examination of a minuscule sample of body tissue beneath a microscope. This tiny specimen can be taken from almost any part of the body or organs where cancer is suspected. I attended the appointment accompanied by my sister and brother-in-law. As I donned the sterile green gown, I felt exposed and vulnerable. The doctor administered local anaesthesia before proceeding. A nurse shielded my eyes with a cloth while another offered her steady grip on my trembling hands. The sensation that followed resembled the piercing agony of a stapler pin as the doctor conducted the procedure twice before meticulously tending to my wounded neck, bandaging it with care.

The ten days that followed were steeped in uncertainty. The wait for the biopsy results was agonizing. Meanwhile, my brother arrived from USA, bearing supplements my mother had dispatched to combat the ominous shadow of cancer. My mother had embarked on her own quest and consulted a holistic doctor who had dispensed a wealth of advice. I surveyed the assortment of exotic remedies and supplements and was engulfed in confusion as I researched each one. After two weeks, my brother and I headed to the hospital to collect the long-awaited reports. Nerves frayed, I asked my brother, "What if it's cancer?" He mumbled something in response; a feeble attempt to soothe my racing mind.

My brother assumed the responsibility of perusing the reports, shielding me from the immediate revelation. However, his countenance spoke volumes, betraying the grim truth before a single word had been uttered. My heart plummeted—I had been hoping against hope for a different outcome. My prayers had fallen on deaf ears.

The next step was to identify the right medical experts. I navigated unfamiliar territory, grappling with a lexicon that included terms like 'oncologist' and 'haematologist.' Thus commenced a series of appointments. The refrain from each specialist bore a semblance of hope— "If God were dispensing afflictions, this one is among the curable." Such words offered solace but couldn't obscure what was coming: chemotherapy, the impending loss of hair and appetite, and all the tribulations ahead. I soon discovered that the first step on this daunting journey entailed a PET scan.

On April 22, I underwent my first PET scan—a Positron Emission Tomography scan—an imaging procedure using radioactive materials to unveil a spectrum of diseases. Physicians rely on this technology to unearth tumours and diagnose heart ailments, neurological disorders, and other conditions. As I bided my time in the waiting area, an empathetic woman offered unsolicited commentary, deeming me 'too young' to be subjected to such tests. Her words unleashed a whirlwind of thought within me. I wondered if everyone in the room had faced a similar battle against cancer. I found myself in the company of two men—a frail elderly gentleman aided by his devoted daughter, and a middle-aged man in his late forties. The realization struck me like a thunderbolt—indeed, I was young. Despite having my own fashion brand, I hadn't made any substantial mark yet. I yearned for a more profound legacy. My life was still devoid of travel experiences and the laughter of children. It felt surreal to sit amidst a bunch of oldies and share the same affliction.

The PET scan was a lengthy affair, starting with the ingestion of 1.5 litres of radioactive water and the insertion of a port line, through which radioactive glucose would flood my system. When my name was called, I entered a chilly room where a colossal machine loomed. With determination, I whispered to it, "We must be friends", hoping it would be generous with me. As I lay down, the mechanical beast went to and fro over me. Warm but agonizing fluids coursed through my upturned hands, immobilizing them for a torturous twenty minutes. Eventually, the ordeal concluded, and I journeyed home alone in a rickshaw, my thoughts consumed by thoughts of how the trajectory of my life had turned.

I had refrained from eating since morning, bracing for the potential collapse that never came. My brother was waiting for me at home. Overwhelmed by fatigue, I surrendered to sleep, awaiting the arrival of the fateful reports. Two days later, they arrived, unequivocally confirming that I harboured active cancer cells on the right side of my neck and armpit, accompanied by lesions on my back. The scan also revealed multiple fibroids—innocent noncancerous growths that typically take residence within the uterine confines. Fortunately, unlike their sinister counterparts, uterine fibroids pose no risk of uterine cancer.

Chapter 2

What Led to Cancer?

As a cancer coach now, I understand that treating cancer requires addressing not only the physical aspect but also delving into the realm of the mind. It has become evident to me that all diseases, including cancer, originate at a mental level before manifesting in the physical body. I was oblivious to this mind-body connection until cancer became an unwelcome guest. I didn't know that stress and depression could lead to such harmful consequences. I had diligently cared for my health through physical activity and healthy lifestyle choices, so being afflicted by such a disease at such a young age shook me to my core.

Questions swirled within me, haunting my thoughts. When did cancer begin developing within my body? Were there subtle signals, symptoms that my body had been trying to convey, signals that I either failed to understand or chose to ignore? My understanding now is that the genesis of cancer can span almost a decade. We all harbour cancer cells within us that bear mutated genes and possess less specialization than normal cells. They operate outside the body's natural order, defying regular growth, division, and cell death cycles. This unchecked proliferation ultimately leads to the emergence of cancer. When the immune system weakens, cancer cells seize the opportunity to multiply faster than the body can defend against. This foundational knowledge led me to understand what factors compromise the immune system. I soon realized that lifestyle choices and stress are pivotal in this delicate balance.

As I contemplated the reasons behind my cancer diagnosis, I retraced my steps to an earlier time, and examined the subtle hints my body had provided. In retrospect, I identified a litany of symptoms that hinted at something being amiss—aches and pains, persistent acidity, unusual bloating, sporadic fever, ceaseless fatigue, restless sleep, and the inexplicable flaking of skin, all indicative of a body struggling to maintain its equilibrium. Regrettably, I had brushed aside these tell-tale signs, attributing them to overwork and pushing my limits. I had held myself to unrealistic expectations—to be a super-achiever and pursue greatness. I did this by taking up challenges constantly in relationships and work.

I now understood my depth of emotion. Each of us has feminine and masculine aspects, which need to be in balance. The left side of our body embodies the feminine, representing qualities such as tenderness, empathy, intuition, and sensuality—yin. Conversely, the right side aligns with the masculine, characterized by attributes like protection, logic, freedom, and direction—yang. It dawned on me that I had habitually overused my masculine energy, which contributed to the cancer's manifestation on the right side of my body, where most of my ailments were found. It left me wondering: How did this pattern begin? Through meditation and inner spiritual work, I unearthed the roots of this imbalance, tracing it back to my constantly fluctuating sense of self-worth.

The two years, marking my separation and impending divorce, had been arduous. Unhappiness and a dark cloud of depression had loomed constantly. Looking back now, it's clear that I had bottled up my emotions to a suffocating degree. My throat chakra had become entirely obstructed, leaving me unable to confront and articulate the agonizing truths about my fractured relationship. Consequently, it was no surprise that my tumour manifested in the region of my neck. A swirling storm of anger, frustration, and fear had taken root within me. The price I paid for this emotional suppression went beyond the confines of my psyche. It found physical expression through the emergence of uterine fibroids, a testament to the wounds inflicted upon my femininity.

Regrettably, the consequences of these afflictions remained veiled until it was far too late. In the aftermath of my failed marriage, I had clung to familiar coping mechanisms, trudging through each day, seeking solace in junk, sugary, and acidic indulgences—a desperate escape from the mundane. My body, craving energy, instinctively reached for caffeine and sugar. Little did I realize that my attempts to stifle the pain created a fertile breeding ground for the insidious cancer cells.

Disease is the body's way of signalling a profound state of 'dis-ease'. The key lies in delving beneath the surface, exploring the root causes rather than merely addressing superficial symptoms. Chronic stress, as I soon learned, wields considerable influence over cancer development by manipulating various physiological processes. It exerts dominion over immune function, inflammation, and DNA repair, all of which are pivotal in the inception and progression of cancer. Psychological stress affects cancer treatment, disrupting adherence to treatment protocols and compromising the body's immune response to therapeutic interventions. Prioritizing stress management during treatment enhances the efficacy of the treatment, ultimately ensuring a higher quality of life for the patient.

Studies now underscore the profound impact of emotions on health. They shed light on the transformative power of happiness, positivity, and gratitude while cautioning against the detrimental effects of negativity and bitterness. Dr Masaru Emoto, a renowned Japanese pseudoscientist, rose to fame with his ground-breaking water experiments chronicled in his book, *The Hidden Messages in Water.*

His experiments involved exposing water to a spectrum of external influences, including music, words, and emotions, followed by freezing the water to observe the resulting ice crystals. Dr Emoto asserted that positive influences gave rise to beautiful, symmetrical crystals, whereas negative ones yielded deformed and unattractive formations.

My cancer diagnosis ignited an unquenchable thirst for knowledge. I was determined to understand every facet of my affliction, equipping myself to confront and combat it on every front. I embarked on an extensive reading journey, devouring everything I could find about cancer to arm myself with the knowledge necessary to wage a multifaceted battle.

A profound misconception about cancer that came to light after my diagnosis was the prevalent belief that it primarily stems from genetic predisposition. In reality, only a tiny fraction, approximately 7-10%, of cancer cases are linked to hereditary factors. Most cancer developments are attributed to the complex interplay between immune responses and many external factors—stress, nutrition, environmental influences, toxins, etc. We encounter two intertwined facets when we delve into cancer genetics.

The first involves genetics inherent to the tumour—the intricate web of genes that are activated or deactivated within the cancerous cells. The second facet pertains to our constitutional genetics, commonly known as germline genetics—the genetic blueprint inherited from our parents, governing our predisposition to various conditions. Most cancers can be traced back to mutations that occur specifically within the group of cells or tissues afflicted by cancer rather than stemming from an inherited genetic susceptibility. This category, accounting for approximately 90% of cancer cases, arises primarily from 'sporadic mutations' with a meagre 5-10% attributed to the genetic inheritance we carry from birth.

Epigenetics is a pivotal field of study, probing the mechanisms by which genes can be selectively activated or silenced reversibly, profoundly impacting their functioning. Specific modifications affect gene expression that determine DNA accessibility to the cellular machinery responsible for gene activation or suppression. These epigenetic marks are not etched in stone; they are influenced by the environment, lifestyle choices, developmental processes, and pre-existing conditions. (https://www.ncbi.nlm.nih.gov/pmc/articles/PMC2515569/- research link)

Aberrations in epigenetic regulation wield substantial influence over various diseases, including cancer. Cancer cells, in particular, exhibit dramatic shifts in their epigenetic landscape when contrasted with normal cells. Alterations in the epigenome unleash a cascade of events, activating oncogenes, which promote uncontrolled cell growth while suppressing the activity of tumour suppressor genes—a sinister choreography that propels the relentless progression of the malignancy.

Chapter 3

The Denial Stage

How does a healthy thirty-four-year-old react when confronted with a cancer diagnosis? The initial response is often disbelief and an inability to comprehend the harsh reality. In my case, denial danced before my eyes during those first few weeks, even as I mechanically moved through the necessary steps ahead.

I clung to the hope that this was a nightmarish jest, a cruel prank that would soon end. I prayed for a return to the normalcy I had known up to that point. Regrettably, I had no choice but to confront the truth. It's an insurmountable challenge to grasp that a life-threatening ailment has befallen one, signalling that something is amiss or that we are 'mortal'. Despite the rational awareness that I now had cancer, my mind stubbornly refused to acknowledge the inconceivable notion that it could happen to me.

The question 'Why me?' loomed larger than life. Why did I have to be the one to endure this? What cosmic injustice had I committed to deserve this cruel twist of fate? I had always taken diligent care of my body and, aside from my grandfather who battled prostate cancer in his 60s—a condition unrelated to Hodgkin's Lymphoma—cancer was absent from my family history. So, what was the rationale behind my being afflicted with this devastating disease?

During those initial days, I remember engaging in fervent conversations with God, my voice raised in questions and accusations regarding the unfortunate hand I had been dealt. There are two types of fighters: those who defy the odds and battle against external forces and those who wage an internal struggle within themselves. I was resolute in my commitment to confront this disease head-on, ready to employ every resource to face whatever trials lay ahead.

Acceptance is a profound concept—one can acknowledge the situation yet remain in denial about the deeper implications. Even as I grappled with the fact that I had cancer, I had not yet truly embraced its presence in my life. 'Why's' and

'How's' continued to swirl within me; I could not understand why cancer had come into *my* life or what it was trying to teach me.

I followed the prescribed protocols almost mechanically—visiting doctors, learning about the intricacies of the disease, and identifying my specific stage in the battle against cancer. I started to acquaint myself with the terminology, educating myself about the facts surrounding my case. My diagnosis placed me at Stage Two, marked by two tumours on my neck, cancer cells lurking in my armpit, and lesions on my back, all clustered on the right side of my body. The slightest movement of my neck caused excruciating pain. Sleep was scarce, and I could only find respite on one side for many nights.

I was far from accepting this disease; I was in combat mode. I resolved to confront cancer on my terms, refusing to follow standard norms and conventional measures. In hindsight, I recognized this as deep-rooted conditioning—a tendency to reject unpleasant things or situations, a habit nurtured since childhood.

Cancer made me think about my life, and I realized it had been a struggle; a ceaseless state of heightened stress response. I had perpetually sought victory and insisted on having things my way. Back in school, I served as House Captain thrice, and relentlessly pursued the top spot. Defeat was an agonizing experience; I distinctly recall shedding tears once when we lost a match. At home, I pursued a solitary existence. I didn't share my thoughts because I believed no one would truly understand me. Cancer served as a mirror, reflecting the subtle patterns I had unwittingly embraced during my formative years that I had carried into adulthood.

Upon deeper reflection, I noticed a recurring pattern—my propensity for choosing arduous and tumultuous paths. In my personal life, I had selected a challenging partner and entered a relationship where I was the relentless pursuer, striving to force a connection that wasn't reciprocated. Professionally, instead of exploring other avenues, I had remained entangled in a stagnant scenario. I had always shied away from openness, and now, I was repeating the same pattern in my approach to battling cancer.

These experiences are catalysts that nudge us towards accepting the need for change in the lifestyle we've adhered to. One must fully accept the situation, the people, and the circumstances as they are, unconditionally. It is what it is. We must learn to adapt and flow with the ever-shifting tides.

From the moment I was diagnosed with cancer, shock rendered me incapable of acceptance. This sentiment lingered for several days; I operated on autopilot. Soon, my ego took over as I couldn't accept that I had fallen victim to something like this. Outwardly, I acknowledged the existence of this disease and the necessary steps I had to take. Internally, I was consumed by a raging denial, plotting various strategies to defeat this affliction. I may not have had a clear-cut plan, but one thing was certain: I was determined to chart a course outside the boundaries of conventional methods, conventional doctors, and the established cancer treatment system.

Chapter 4
The Inevitable Testing Stage

The phase of testing that follows when cancer is suspected is undoubtedly one of the most gruelling ordeals—a trial not just for the body but for the mind as well. During this time, thoughts run rampant, often conjuring the darkest possible outcomes. These tests are painful; they devour your time, and cast a shadow of despair. Waiting to learn the truth is pure torment. You find yourself unable to relax, trapped in constant anticipation until you know what is happening in your body.

Unfortunately, there's no avoiding this harrowing process; it's the only path to uncover the precise nature of the problem. I was tested across all facets of my life during this time: health, relationships, career, spirituality, finances, and home. And I faced these trials in solitude.

Typically, one has a loved one or a family member by their side, or at least a mentor who can guide one through it. However, I had always been disinclined to discuss challenging matters. This reluctance to openly address issues was a by-product of an upbringing that shaped me into a lone wolf. In hindsight, I would have made better decisions had I approached things more objectively. Irrational emotions can lead us down the wrong path.

Formulating my treatment plan was no easy feat—choosing the right doctor, deciding which approaches to incorporate, and navigating the labyrinth of advice from countless sources, left me utterly bewildered. I couldn't think clearly enough to discern whom to trust and whom to question. My life had been upended; my health was deteriorating, my marriage had crumbled, and some friendships had disintegrated. It was an eye-opening revelation to discover that certain friends only showed up in my life when it suited them. I had experienced this in the past: relationships where I had offered a sympathetic ear to their grievances, but when I needed support, they turned away. This had left me perpetually seeking validation from others, stemming from certain childhood triggers. However, cancer served as a teacher, driving home the lesson that I can and must establish boundaries, particularly with those close to my heart. I had to pull down the shutters on my retail store and adapt to a home-based work routine. My financial situation was precarious, and I was compelled to handle every aspect of my life independently. When I think back, I can't quite fathom from where I mustered the strength to plough on.

I probably inherited this trait to endure from my mother, despite our complex relationship. She displays unwavering determination in all her endeavours, a quality I had unwittingly absorbed. Witnessing her constant struggle at home, whether in her approach to raising us or her relationship with my father, profoundly impacted me. I felt a deep affection for my mother, even as I watched her endure challenges without fully embracing the present and the simple joys around her. Now, I could understand the lasting impression it left on me. When I entered into marriage, I carried with me an expectation of adversity, a belief that life is meant to be an eternal struggle—a misconception I've since discarded. In hindsight, it's evident that we choose these patterns;

they reside in our subconscious mind. We attract individuals vibrating on similar frequencies. Regardless of circumstances, we are responsible for our health and lives.

The PET scan was the worst experience. I had to drink sugary, radioactive water dosed according to my weight and height. Subsequently, a painful intravenous injection was administered within the imposing confines of a huge scanning apparatus. I lay immobile, my hands suspended above my head, which was excruciating due to the pain that gripped my entire right side, from the armpit to my neck and hand. Each time I was subjected to this procedure, surrounded by fellow patients, my mind wove a tapestry of vivid and unsettling narratives. Would I eventually succumb and be rendered helpless and disabled, my organs ravaged beyond repair? These thoughts, unfettered and unrestrained, haunted my consciousness. While Hodgkin's Lymphoma primarily targets the immune system, I remained ignorant of the potential collateral damage it could inflict.

Chapter 5
The Blame Game

The easiest thing to do when something goes wrong is to blame others and external circumstances, and shield oneself from taking responsibility. I found myself in this trap. I directed my resentment towards my failed marriage and my ex-husband, pouring out my anguish to him over the phone, my tears mirroring my despair. In those moments, I fervently wished that the events between us had unfolded differently. I repeatedly voiced the belief that I was in this dire situation solely because of him, that the wounds he had inflicted had somehow transmuted into the cancer coursing through me. And, perhaps, harshest of all, I turned the blame inward, chastising myself for the poor choices that had led me to this juncture.

Anger coursed through me, not just towards myself, but towards others. I was even angry with God. Why was I the one burdened with suffering? What had I done to deserve this cruel fate? I was on the precipice of embarking on a solitary journey, a path that was scary enough. On top of everything else, I was burdened with this horrifying illness without knowing how long it would persist or what lingering consequences I would bear. My emotions choked me, leaving me incapable of baring my soul to anyone. My turmoil was a tempest of anger, guilt, and shame. I blamed every conceivable facet of my life, from people to circumstances, seeking an outlet for my anguish.

As I strived to understand the origins of cancer, I realized it could be a result of festering resentment, enduring grief, and profound hurt, of which I had my fair share. Negative thoughts bubbled up incessantly, with blame extending to my parents, particularly directed to my mother. Our relationship had been strained since childhood when I had listened to her but resented many of her decisions on my behalf. For instance, I had wanted to pursue higher studies in art at Baroda. I had even secured admission, but my mother had opposed the idea. I had to finish my college education in Ujjain and study subjects I had little interest in. I hadn't even forgiven her for this when she began pressuring me to get married. When I was nineteen, she began scouting for potential suitors, a decision I found utterly baffling. It sparked a rebellion; I yearned to explore the world, discover myself, acquire an education, and travel. However, I felt trapped, reduced to an object whose sole purpose was marriage and everything that followed.

This experience inflicted lasting scars on my self-esteem as the first man I met rejected me. I was too young and lacked knowledge of what to look for in a partner or even how to hold a meaningful conversation. My mother was keen that I marry sooner rather than later, believing I would 'settle down'. This created a distance between us, and it took me considerable time to release the anger I had harboured towards her for these choices.

In time, my mother's stance towards me began to evolve, particularly after I completed college and voiced my desire to move to Mumbai to pursue a fashion course. My decision to relocate garnered little support from others around me, but my mother stepped up. She arranged my accommodation for the first few months and accompanied me to ensure my comfort. She played a crucial role in organizing my finances and aiding me in my education and self-discovery. It's safe to say that my relationship with her was marked by highs and lows—a curious blend of warmth and coolness. During my time in Bombay, my mother patiently taught me how to navigate the bustling city streets, including the art of crossing the road. It seemed absurd that I harboured a fear of something as mundane as crossing the street in Mumbai. However, beneath the surface, a simmering anger remained nestled in my heart, an unresolved issue I carried with me for a long time.

Diseases often find their origins in the past. Cancer, in particular, can take up to two decades to manifest. Cancer lurks silently within our bodies, evading detection through asymptomatic phases. This covert stage underscores the importance of regular screenings. However, certain cancers, called symptomatic cancers, manifest tell-tale symptoms early. Timely diagnosis is vital, as it paves the way for successful treatment and offers the reassurance that the source of distressing symptoms may be benign.

A Stanford University School of Medicine study published in the *Science Translational Medicine* journal provides evidence that malignant tumours may grow undetected in the body for a decade or more before being detected by sophisticated blood tests. This emphasizes the urgent need to identify and clinically validate more sensitive biological markers (biomarkers) that can detect tiny cancers in the body before they grow large enough to become high-risk.

The existing societal framework must change, particularly in how we nurture and educate our children. Parents must be equipped with comprehensive strategies for raising their children holistically. Before bringing new life into the world, parents should be emotionally, mentally, spiritually, and physically prepared to foster the growth of healthy children.

Traditional educational institutions often fail to provide the necessary tools for handling emotions and life's practical challenges. Children must be educated in practical life skills that encompass navigating adversity, nurturing mental wellbeing, understanding nutrition, and developing emotional resilience. The prevalence of mental health issues among today's children is alarming, with rising instances of illness, aggression, and challenging behaviour.

I've come to understand that most cancers are a by-product of our lifestyles, shaped by our choices in processed food, managing thoughts, and interacting with our environment. This should not be taken lightly. While interacting with numerous cancer patients, I noticed the common threads binding them—fear, confusion, guilt, and other emotions ensnared within their cells. The societal norms we inherit during our formative years influence our personalities and behaviours, often leaving us ill-equipped to confront life's challenges. There is no definite right or wrong, and our approaches to managing emotions and wellbeing are diverse. Emotions find their dwelling places within our organs and cellular structures, and life-altering events such as cancer can catalyse dramatic transformations. Some individuals emerge embittered, while others embark on journeys of self-discovery and introspection.

Chapter 6
The Confusion Stage

Half-baked knowledge is futile and potentially dangerous when fighting a life-altering challenge like cancer. No one has an answer as to why cancer occurs. The time spent consulting doctors and diving into the intricacies of the disease was taxing. Everyone echoed the same sentiment—I should be thankful because, among the diseases one could get, this cancer was relatively treatable. Did this provide genuine hope? Not particularly.

Research indicates that individuals above 40 without any history of blood pressure, heart ailments, or other health conditions constitute a mere 1% of the population—a demographic I still found myself part of! So, the question reverberating in my mind was whether there was another path, an alternative to conventional treatment. My quest to explore different approaches became all-consuming. I joined various social media groups to understand people's cancer journeys while conducting exhaustive internet research. My plan was simple: give myself six months to pursue my methods and then decide on the next steps. I held a somewhat eccentric belief that I could heal without medication, influenced mainly by my mother, a Sujok therapist.

My mother's unwavering faith had led her to meet numerous individuals who had cured themselves, naturally. She had her own story, having conquered acute back problems, varicose veins, and arthritis. I remember her being bedridden when I was in the fourth grade. She had to undergo traction for her back, her leg was suspended for ten days, and painful antibiotics became a part of her daily routine. Her resilience left an indelible mark on me as I navigated my studies independently, seeking occasional assistance from my cousins. When traction proved insufficient, my dad and she embarked on a month-long journey to Indore for holistic acupressure and acupuncture treatments. She returned a transformed woman, her pain dissipated, and a renewed sense of vitality coursing through her. From then on, she immersed herself in studying natural remedies, harbouring an aversion to allopathic meds. To this day, she leads a medication-free life and helps others discover an alternative path to wellness and a new way to live.

We explored alternative treatments as a joint venture, though we had little prior experience. We ventured into Ayurveda, naturopathy, gluten-free diets, massage, ozone therapy, and yoga. Surrounded by people who had traversed similar paths in their cancer journeys, each with their unique approach, I was inundated with multiple perspectives.

I did not give up dairy because as a vegetarian I worried about where I would get the necessary protein and calcium. I was brought up on the notion that milk is good for health and had been gulping down three glasses of milk since childhood. It was hard for me to imagine giving up any dairy products, especially cheese, ice creams, favourite desserts and various yogurts. I couldn't imagine cooking without ghee or not finishing my meals with buttermilk. I didn't know what I could replace these comfort foods with as I didn't have a mentor to guide me. There was a great emotional resistance, which was nothing short of bewildering for me and my body.

In retrospect, I realized I was taking various steps without fully comprehending the underlying principles. I witnessed my condition improve, indicating that some of the treatments were working. However, in my mind I was still grappling with my deepest fears: the need for forgiveness and the challenge of acceptance. Looking back, my actions during this phase seemed more like a rebellion against cancer than well-informed, proactive choices.

Deciding to take the unconventional path was intimidating. I was in a peculiar mental state as I was still I the process of separating from my husband. I needed to distance myself from the world, avoiding explanations to extended family and friends. I had no desire to make my illness public knowledge. I didn't want to be pitied. I recall a close friend shedding tears upon hearing the news, and her reaction made me feel worse. I shared my diagnosis with only a handful of people because I wanted to figure out everything independently.

Since childhood, my subconscious urged me towards self-reliance. I believed I had to navigate life's challenges on my own. I was convinced no one could truly understand me. This communication issue persisted as I grew older, leading me to harbour emotions and grievances, particularly regarding what people said or did to me. Letting go of such feelings was a long process. I spun intricate narratives based on their words and the emotions they evoked. I now understand that these reactions stemmed from insecurity, a reluctance to prioritize my wellbeing, and a lack of emotional self-care. I had always been a giver, whether with friends or other relationships. I tended to give even more when deeply attached, but my expectations from those to whom I gave my all became a stumbling block.

Chapter 7
Doing the Best I Can

I was dealing with Stage Two cancer, a condition that, while serious, wasn't an immediate threat to life. However, like many allopathic doctors, mine were far from pleased with my decision to explore natural healing methods. They asked me to reconsider, emphasizing lymphoma's aggressive nature that could lead it to invade other organs in my body. However, I wasn't prepared to grapple with the repercussions of conventional treatment mentally and physically. I needed time to make sense of the whirlwind that had swept through my life. So, I resolved to alter my daily routine and dietary habits. I devoted my time to understanding the world of natural healing and treatments, determined to give them a fair chance.

My mother had long been immersed in natural healing through her Sujok practice (Sujok Therapy is a healing methodology based on Acupressure, and is a simple method that produces highly effective results). She was adamant that I avoid allopathic protocols, explaining that numerous individuals had successfully cured themselves through alternative methods. Her unwavering belief in this approach played a pivotal role in guiding my journey towards understanding this mode of healing.

In an unexpected way, this break was a blessing to me. It allowed me to gain a deeper understanding of my life and myself. I had always been on the move, constantly striving to achieve something. My cancer diagnosis forced me to halt and engage in profound introspection. Despite the doctors' ominous warnings, I took a leap of faith. For six to seven months, I distanced myself from the influence of others, disregarding their opinions and suggestions. I made myself the focal point and dedicated my focus to self-healing.

This journey was a mixed bag, filled with valuable lessons. Shutting others out taught me to stop seeking validation from external sources. Instead, I turned inward to find peace. It gave me the time to choose whether I wanted to continue being the person I had always been. During this time, I built walls to see who genuinely cared for me and who would cross bridges for me. The results were eye-opening. It served as a filtration process, helping me distinguish my true friends and family—those I could genuinely rely on—from those who were transient in my life. I harbour no ill will towards anyone, but I've realized that some people enter your life merely to test you and impart important life lessons. Good or bad, these experiences contribute to your personal growth, if you can learn from them. I used to get upset, agitated, and frustrated, always seeking answers to why someone had behaved in a certain way. The lack of answers always left me hurting. However, cancer taught me to accept that there are situations and people beyond our control and to let go.

This was particularly challenging for an empath like me—someone who feels the pain of others deeply, is sensitive, intuitive, and prone to becoming easily overwhelmed and anxious. Letting go was never my forte, and achieving balance often felt hard. I had to learn these essential life lessons the hard way! I won't deny there are still days when people's actions affect me, but when I reflect on what I've endured, I can summon the strength to regain my composure.

Cancer has the potential to make you stronger if you permit yourself to view it from various angles. That's why I now advise all my patients not to label this experience as inherently good or bad. Let it run its course, and you'll eventually glean the wisdom it offers. You'll come to understand what it seeks to teach you.

I made a conscious choice to abstain from immediate conventional treatment. Instead, I invested time in comprehending cancer's impact on me, and I don't regret that decision. Many people criticized me, deeming it a waste of time and a delay in treatment. They couldn't perceive the wisdom I gained. People enjoy commenting on others' lives and journeys but rarely fathom their internal battles. I don't take their opinions to heart anymore. I evaluate whose perspectives truly matter and deserve consideration. No one knows your journey better than you do; the same applies to your body. No one understands it better than you. Developing a profound connection with your body is essential. Most of us merely use it, but as you delve deeper into its intricacies, your intuition will grow stronger and become a trusted friend. You'll then naturally gravitate towards choices that are in its best interest.

Chapter 8
Turning Point

When I decided to forego conventional treatments, it was a turning point, requiring me to confront my cancer head-on and make substantial lifestyle changes. One of the first and most challenging changes I made was to eliminate sugar from my diet, as I had learned that sugar is a source of nourishment for cancer cells. I realized I was addicted to sugar. I craved something sweet after every meal and found myself drawn to sugary foods. Little did I know that these cravings were linked to certain nutritional deficiencies within my body. Overhauling this aspect of my life was the toughest challenge. I removed all chocolates, desserts, Indian sweets, and white sugar from my kitchen, determined to survive without them. Additionally, I decided to bid farewell to processed foods, which meant I practically stopped dining out. The chips, colas, and fried snacks that were once my regular indulgences became a thing of the past. I even refrained from visiting grocery stores and my favourite coffee shops.

My research enlightened me about the inflammatory effects of gluten, as most wheat products contain genetically modified organisms (GMOs). Consequently, I switched to organic foods and stopped drinking milk, which meant giving up my beloved tea and coffee. I couldn't help but wonder how I would manage. Studies show that dairy products promote inflammation and contain casein, a carcinogenic protein. This prompted me to examine the source of the milk I consumed. Nonetheless, I continued to incorporate ghee and paneer derived from the milk of organic grass-fed cows in my diet, as they were exceptional protein sources.

I slowly introduced supplements into my daily routine as well. One addition was Essiac tea from the USA, a herbal blend discovered by a nurse working with cancer patients. It is renowned for its cancer-fighting properties. Flaxseed oil, rich in Omega-3 fatty acids that help regulate hormones, became a staple. Vitamin C was crucial in boosting my immune system, while turmeric, known for its anti-cancer properties, was recommended by a naturopath.

One unconventional treatment I underwent was ozone therapy, which involved the direct application of ozone to the tumour site, where it enters through the skin. After doing a G6PD test, which measures the protein that helps red blood cells function properly, I started with a low-dose of ozone through rectal, nose, and ears. Once the body tolerates it well enough, it is given through an IV. The theory is that cancer cells cannot live in an oxygenated environment as they are anaerobic. Although ozone therapy was relatively new and not widely known then, I read testimonials and met patients who had benefitted from it. Ozone therapy enhances oxygenation in the body, fortifies the immune system, and inhibits the growth of cancer cells.

https://www.ncbi.nlm.nih.gov/pmc/articles/PMC442111/

I wholeheartedly embraced Ayurveda, incorporating various herbs and therapies to aid my battle against cancer. Transitioning to this new way of life required a significant adjustment, completely altering my routine from what it was before. Due to the biopsy on my neck, there was a minuscule hole, and my Ayurvedic therapist recommended applying warm compresses. One day, to my astonishment, the tumour emerged from the biopsy site. It felt like my body was expelling toxicity and the pent-up emotions I had harboured. Following the tumour's emergence, the area would often bleed, especially at night when it experienced pressure. I would wake up with bloodstains on my neck and the upper part of my T-shirt. Fearing to touch the tumour and its surroundings, I concealed it beneath neck scarves whenever I ventured outside.

I adopted the yogic way of life as well. I incorporated yoga practices, focussing on controlled breathing and pranayama as complementary therapies to aid my battle against cancer. During a private yoga class, I discovered my breathing was shallow and incorrect. My instructor identified that I was deflating my abdomen instead of inflating it when breathing in. I soon realized that years of poor posture from a semi-sedentary lifestyle had rendered my lungs inefficient. My habit of slouching and compressing my lungs had reduced their effectiveness. We typically utilize only 30% of our total lung capacity.

Ayurveda introduced me to the concept of enemas, which sounded so unappealing. Nevertheless, armed with a wealth of information, I decided to try it. The enema process entails introducing fluids through the anal tract into the intestines, requiring one to retain it briefly before promptly heading to the restroom. Although I had reservations at the outset, I learned from therapies like Gerson's and others that coffee enemas in particular, can eliminate circulating toxins and partially metabolized substances by dilating the bile ducts and detoxifying the liver. Ayurvedic medicine aligns with this notion, explaining that the liver regenerates and replaces itself every three months. Coffee enemas assist in flushing out toxic bile and its salts, liberating the body from harmful waste products of metabolism, such as protein derivatives, toxic-bound nitrogen, amino acids, and coagulated clumps. By purging these substances, the body is safeguarded against self-poisoning.

https://www.cancerresearchuk.org/about-cancer/treatment/complementary-alternative-therapies/individual-therapies/yoga

I diligently practiced Kapalabhati a hundred times with intervals of Anulom Vilom and Bhramari Pranayama half an hour every morning and evening. I incorporated a thirty-minute daily walk into my routine and two weekly lymphatic massages. Additionally, I embraced high doses of Vitamin C. After three or four months of unwavering commitment to these practices, the C-Reactive Protein levels, a blood test marker for cancer, dropped from 32 to within the normal range. Curiously, my doctors never monitored these tests, even though they reflected the inflammatory response in my blood. I couldn't contain my joy at the results of my efforts. I thought to myself, "Wow, it's working! Should I continue with what I'm doing?" Overall, I felt incredibly optimistic and satisfied with this transition. It was as if I had unlocked the secret to wellness. The ego boost from witnessing the efficacy of these methods validated my treatment choices, reinvigorated my energy levels, and contributed to the shrinking of the tumour, which was truly astonishing.

Although I remained mentally focussed and in a better emotional space, the pain on the right side of my neck persisted. I still couldn't lift my hand and found it uncomfortable to sleep on the right side, although the intensity of the pain had diminished compared to earlier. I showed my reports to Dr Mill, who was overseeing my ozone therapy, which had demonstrated success in numerous cancer cases. She expressed her satisfaction with my progress, but I understood that the battle was far from over. Until my PET scans returned with clean results, I needed to persist with my rigorous efforts.

Still in my self-imposed cocoon, I limited my interactions with others and channelled my focus inward. During this time, I acquired a deeper understanding of self-love and self-care. I realized that I had wasted considerable energy on worrying about what others thought of me, ruminating over past mistakes, absorbing the hurt inflicted by others, and nurturing unrealistic expectations from life. This encompassed all the regrets and decisions that had led me to my current situation in the first place.

Coming right off my toxic marriage and before I had any chance to restart my life, cancer had a massive impact on my mental wellbeing. I had underestimated the toll it would take and the time required for full acceptance. However, once I accepted it, I waged an internal battle against cancer. The struggle was constant within me, and summoning the mental fortitude to rise each day, adhere to my challenging new routine, and confront the world demanded every ounce of my resilience. Thus, as I progressed toward recovery and felt better than when I embarked on this journey, my confidence soared, and I found myself in a positive state of mind. The pressing question now loomed: *What additional measures could I adopt to obliterate this cancer threat? How could I attain complete health and fitness and make a triumphant comeback?*

Chapter 9

Going Downhill

My journey had been progressing well, and I held hope for my recovery. However, in November 2016, a sudden and alarming development shook me up. I noticed the emergence of another small tumour from the biopsy site, leaving me baffled and frightened. If everything was on track, then why had this new challenge surfaced? Once again, I managed the bloodstains and sought ozone treatment. Some people said it was a positive sign indicating the release of impurities, but the sight of it was far from comforting, both for my eyes and my mind. I concealed the tumour from prying eyes beneath a scarf whenever I ventured outside. My wardrobe now consisted of an array of scarves in various colours that became my signature style. I often donned palazzo pants paired with loose T-shirts, a scarf draped around my neck, and my jhola bag.

My second disappointment arrived shortly after discovering that my CRP and ESR levels were rising. This disconcerting development left me anxious. It seemed like the ground was about to crumble beneath me. Rejecting conventional therapy in favour of a holistic approach had been a gamble, and now my ego was taking a beating. I had believed I had the cancer under control, knew what needed to be done, and could conquer it. But suddenly, it all came crashing down like a house of cards. I had wanted to prove to the world that I was in control, that I could defy fate and shape my destiny. Little did I realize that sometimes, relentless resistance is not the answer.

I had been fighting cancer like a boss with unyielding determination, thinking I had it all figured out. However, my body was exhibiting signs of revolt. My ability to digest food had deteriorated, leading to weight loss, disrupted eating and sleeping patterns, and exacerbated pain. By mid-December, I began experiencing bouts of vomiting and severe acidity. The mere act of eating triggered these episodes. I travelled to my hometown, Ujjain, where I met with cousins and extended family. Sleep eluded me due to relentless back pain, forcing me to seek relief through hot-water compresses. A coldness enveloped me, and the vomiting continued after every meal. It was a disheartening experience, and I could sense my health deteriorating day by day. Each day, I looked into the mirror and beheld a reflection of disease, sadness, and fear, It was as if the vital force within me was draining out.

Doubts began to cloud the minds of those around me even as I questioned the path I had chosen. Fear of failure now gripped me tightly, and I was determined not to falter. But my body was screaming for help. Perhaps I had erred in my approach, or my efforts were insufficient. My mother sought advice from various sources and acquired medicines, some with cow urine and others with herbs. I was experimenting extensively and placing tremendous pressure on myself. At one point, I felt I was pursuing too many conflicting strategies. While I loosely followed Gerson's Therapy, I deviated from it significantly, formulating my own concoctions and combining various elements without guidance. January 2017 proved agonizing. The constant pain in my neck persisted, impeding my ability to walk properly. I summoned extra strength to fulfil necessary tasks, yet I struggled with inadequate sleep, overwhelming fatigue, and further weight loss.

During that time, information was scarce regarding steps to combat cancer naturally. No one provided me with a definitive roadmap for the next steps, or perhaps I was not looking in the right places. Nevertheless, I had to take action, even though I felt trapped. My unwavering persistence and stubbornness allowed me to continue despite the relentless pain.

Chapter 10
Finding Acceptance

From a young age, my family were dedicated followers of our Master. His guidance was our compass, be it on matters of spiritual growth or significant life decisions. Personal issues, business choices, marriages, and any other challenges were first discussed with him. Despite enduring numerous trials and tribulations, our family rarely succumbed to bitterness. Perhaps, on occasion, there was a hint of it, but everyone faced their hardships with remarkable resilience. From uncles to aunts to cousins, every family member encountered their share of trials, acknowledged them, and ultimately conquered them. It was a difficult journey for all, but no one truly shattered. It was faith that provided the unwavering strength to persevere. I had nurtured a profound belief system rooted in the teachings of Sant Math. However, when cancer entered my life, I questioned everything, even my faith.

I grappled with anger, convinced that I didn't deserve this ordeal—I kept asking why I had to endure such suffering. Answers to such questions don't come swiftly; they slowly emerge over time. During a visit to my hometown in January 2017, I accompanied my parents to meet our Master. All they sought from him was guidance on what to do. His response was simple and direct: "Follow the doctors' advice, and you will recover."

I wept silently before him, my voice stifled by emotion. He too had confronted and overcome cancer. He reassured me, "You'll regain your hair," pointing to his beard as if he sensed my dread of losing hair. On the drive home after meeting him, I sobbed uncontrollably as if my ego had been shattered. In the days that followed, regardless of who came to visit me, all I could do was cry. I have no recollection of when I returned to Mumbai; it's as if it occurred in a dream.

Subsequently, the first step we took was to identify a doctor who could provide us with proper guidance and repeat the PET scan. We opted for Raheja Hospital, where we received the disheartening news that my cancer had progressed to Stage Three. Although the lesions on my back had vanished, indicating that some measures had proven effective, new tumours had emerged on my right side, above the lungs. This explained the persistent vomiting I had been experiencing. The doctors admonished me for delaying my treatment and questioned why I hadn't sought help earlier.

It's challenging to convey the immense fear that hangs over your head when you receive a diagnosis of this magnitude. Doctors encounter numerous patients everyday and become accustomed to such situations but for each patient it's their first encounter with this reality. Naturally, they need time to come to terms with it and decide upon the best course of action. I had a mere two weeks before the treatment began, during which I had to accept that I needed to follow the conventional medical route. During those two weeks, I tried to look at cancer from a different perspective like it had come to teach me some valuable life lessons. I tried to figure out what my cancer was trying to show me.

First, I had to release my fear and learn to live in the present. It was exceedingly difficult not to dwell on the uncertainties of the future. I embarked on an educational journey, absorbing everything about the forthcoming treatment, its potential onslaught on my body, and the ensuing side effects, and explored strategies to mitigate them. My two primary concerns centred around hair loss and the impact of cancer on my fertility. I delved into comprehensive research and bombarded my doctors with questions on how to safeguard both. I recall sitting in the doctor's office, eagerly seeking information on fertility preservation. While no guarantees or specific timelines were provided, I was told that hormonal injections administered before chemotherapy could help protect my ovaries.

The chemotherapy regimen I was prescribed was ABVD-t, comprising doxorubicin hydrochloride (Adriamycin), Bleomycin Sulphate, Vinblastine Sulphate, and Dacarbazine. The potential side effects included nausea, fatigue, constipation, or diarrhea. There was a chance this could affect my heart, lead to fluctuations in blood pressure, and trigger headaches. The doctor gave me a comprehensive list of potential conditions I might encounter and an array of medications to address them. It seemed somewhat perplexing, but I decided not to question the doctor's expertise.

Accepting cancer is an intense process. It transcends surface-level acknowledgment and extends deep into one's core. True acceptance calls for a readiness to assume responsibility for the illness and to undertake any necessary measures to overcome it, while striving to comprehend its root cause. After relentlessly battling it for so long, I finally assumed responsibility for my journey.

Chapter 11
Going with the Flow

Letting go is an integral component of the acceptance process, but the phrase "Let go" is often used without a clear understanding of what it entails. Through my journey, I've recognized that relinquishing control is the most challenging aspect of letting go. Humans possess an inherent desire to maintain control, whether in our expectations of our partners, our wishes for how our children should behave, or our preference for temperature-controlled environments. We even domesticate and train our pets.

I'm not suggesting that we should let go of everything; however, there are some things we should release—our thoughts, inhibitions, fears, and the need to conform to others' opinions. I was active and engaged at school, but I often felt a sense of melancholy at home. I'd immerse myself in daydreams, and solitude became my refuge. There were moments when I couldn't relate to others. I turned to dancing, writing, and music to cope with these emotions. My tendency to conceal my feelings and avoid open communication took root. I had observed resistance to difficult conversations at home, and while I didn't fully comprehend it then, these behaviours continued to impact me in adulthood.

When I interact with cancer patients now, particularly women, I notice similar patterns in many of them—keeping their emotions bottled and trying to solve problems on their own. This confirms my belief that the body stores emotions that ultimately manifest as diseases. While I don't claim that it is the sole determinant, it undeniably plays a significant role in cancer development.

I often wish that schools included counselling sessions for children. There's an emphasis on children adhering to certain behavioural norms and on academic achievements, but it often ignores their emotional wellbeing. In my case, habits established during childhood became deep-rooted. One of my self-sabotaging tendencies was the inclination to avoid speaking up. I recall an incident from my early years when I approached my parents with a request, only to witness them engaged in a heated argument. For some inexplicable reason, this impacted me, leading me to believe that I wasn't important. This belief lingered for many years until I discovered the concept of healing one's inner child—an aspect of the subconscious that retains past wounds from childhood. An inner child can be shaped by emotional or physical abuse, bullying, or even seemingly innocuous moments that a child interprets as traumatic. I embarked on a journey to become my own parent, revisiting my past and providing myself with the love I found lacking.

Despite living in a joint family with two siblings and six cousins, my thought process often diverged. I gravitated towards solitude and sought solace in journaling about my emotions and thoughts. I had little inclination for family gossip or conforming to prescribed behaviour. I struggled to articulate my desires and needs, a trait that later caused complications in my relationships and marriage. I often opted for silence to avoid conflict and maintain harmony, oblivious to the harm it was causing me. This inclination toward people-pleasing is a common trait among many girls. I constantly tried to be amiable and conform to my husband's expectations. If I disliked something, I found it hard to express my concerns. I believed I was responsible for mending the relationship, as I had chosen my partner. Gradually, my suppressed emotions began to manifest as disease symptoms, as I unwittingly clung to anger, regret, and resentment for an extended period.

Truly sitting with yourself and relinquishing things that are part of your emotional baggage is a formidable task that demands effort and courage. Letting go is a nuanced process, far more challenging than casual conversations about it suggest. So, what exactly do we need to release? First and foremost, we must relinquish the illusion of control over how people behave and control the outcomes of our lives. Simply performing good deeds, we should allow results to unfold in their own time, favourable or unfavourable. Our constant desire for immediate answers is a source of significant suffering. I firmly believe impatience lies at the core of much of our pain. The most formidable aspect of letting go was releasing my grip on the outcome of my battle with cancer. Letting go is an ongoing practice, and the journey is far from linear. Some days, it works splendidly, while on other days, it falters. The initial step is to continually remind yourself that you have everything you need in the present moment and express gratitude. It involves experimenting with oneself, identifying what challenges you, and developing a personal mantra to live by. This process, though arduous, is essential for growth, whether one confronts cancer or navigates the everyday complexities of life. Although it would undoubtedly be preferable without the added burden of cancer.

In my journey, I began by releasing the fear of what chemotherapy would do to my body. Then, I needed to let go of my apprehensions about the future, including thoughts of my mortality or the prospect of contracting other illnesses, even additional cancers. Gradually, I coaxed myself into a state of acceptance, allowing me to live each day and address one issue at a time. Deep-seated fears and elements of consciousness cannot be discarded overnight; it's a deliberate, ongoing process. I faced a pivotal choice: succumb to worry or rise above it to carve out my desired life.

I chose the latter path, which made my journey more manageable. I directed my energies toward preparing my mind to confront the side effects of chemotherapy. Releasing fear and other burdens created space for other thoughts and pursuits. Resentment and anger act as live electrical wires, burning you each time you touch them. Shedding unnecessary clutter from my life helped me experience freedom, and I found it easier to relinquish feelings of resentment. My entire focus shifted to overcoming cancer, and I was ready to take whatever measure were necessary to safeguard and improve my wellbeing. Prioritizing oneself and one's health is paramount. However, it's essential to choose your battles wisely. This is a good time not to attempt to resolve everyone's issues. It's okay to decline that phone call, limit communication with your family, or seek minimal assistance if you prefer to confront matters independently. This doesn't imply a lack of care for others; it's about understanding how to strike a balance that aligns with your body and mind's requirements in battling the disease.

As a cancer patient, I discovered that many emotions reside in one's mind, and receiving a cancer diagnosis can lead to depression. When excessive introspection revolves around life's perceived wrongs, it exacerbates anxiety. By letting go of excessive thoughts and their mental burden, I felt lighter and better equipped to face the impending battle with my illness. I made a firm decision: my divorce could wait, my friends could wait, my family could wait, my clients could wait.

I couldn't help but ponder if there might be a comprehensive, integrated system capable of alleviating this suffering, something conventional treatments often neglect. Research has unveiled a connection between cancer and stress. While not everyone experiences this connection, retaining fear or resentment can contribute to anxiety. For my own wellbeing, I resolved to forgive and forget everything that had transpired in my life—the childhood abuse I endured, the physical assaults inflicted by my ex-husband, and the betrayal of people around me—enabling me to embark on a journey of complete healing.

Chapter 12
Living in the Present

"Live in the present, don't worry about the future or the past" is a well-known piece of advice, but it's challenging to put it into practice. How can a cancer patient, or anyone else for that matter, stop overthinking? During my chemotherapy treatments, I delved into meditation and visualization. I cultivated a mental image where the chemotherapy exclusively targeted cancer cells, leaving my healthy cells untouched. My days were filled with listening to guided meditation, satsangs, shlokas, and more. In this process, I unearthed the incredible power of concentration and living in the moment without fixating on outcomes. My long-standing habits of overthinking and procrastination began to dissipate.

I adopted a day-by-day approach, both before and after chemotherapy. Beyond planning for the immediate hour post-treatment, I refrained from dwelling on the future. For the remainder of the day, my focus remained on recuperation and nurturing my mental wellbeing. I invested time reading books on nutrition, cancer, and healing, ultimately recognizing the significant role lifestyle plays in cancer. I was astounded by the stories of individuals who had faced even harsher cancer journeys than mine, who had persevered, and were now leading purposeful lives.

During this period, there were instances when I genuinely forgot I had cancer. My mind had become so unburdened and light. I would engage in light-hearted banter with the nurses at Lilavati Hospital in Bandra, where I received my treatment. They often remarked on my jovial and pleasant disposition, which, in turn, brightened my spirits. This time was invaluable for teaching me how to let go of constant worry—something I had long struggled with. I began relishing moments spent with my parents who had returned from the USA to accompany me during treatment. We watched television shows like Indian Idol, Shark Tank, and documentaries on the History Channel.

When I was a child, a family doctor had referred to me as a 'worrier' due to my perpetually sweaty palms and cold feet. They were physiological signs of an underactive thyroid and overworked adrenals despite my normal blood markers. As a holistic coach today, I emphasize the importance of assessing blood markers and considering the body's symptoms in evaluating health. Generic blood marker ranges can be misleading; our bodily symptoms must be considered. The family doctor suggested that my nervous system was in a state of hyperactivity. I didn't fully grasp this concept then, but I started connecting the dots during my treatment. I realized I had perpetually been in a state of 'fight or flight.' I was reacting to my past, fixating on what had gone wrong, how I could have done things differently, and how nothing seemed to be in my control. Symptomatically, my immune system was compromised, manifesting in perpetual nasal congestion, low energy levels, heightened reactivity, and chronic overthinking. Some of these tendencies still linger, but now I'm conscious of them.

There was constant turmoil in my mind because I was unhappy with my circumstances—a pattern that persisted since childhood. I harboured ambitions that remained unrealized. In my youth, I yearned to become an air hostess, not merely for the independence it promised but as a means to assert control over my life. I sought to escape my small hometown, believing it would hinder my growth and give me an opportunity to interact with intriguing individuals. My heart brimmed with wild, adventurous spirit, craving travel and offbeat encounters. I had reservations about my family situation. While we enjoyed a comfortable life in a beautiful home with modern amenities, I felt confined, unable to escape and pursue my dreams. My college years were spent in a place that did not resonate with me, and it rankled.

In hindsight, I now understand that everything has a purpose, and true happiness doesn't hinge solely on accomplishments but on cherishing the blessings we possess. I wish I had understood this before distancing myself from my true self. In my younger days, I yearned for answers, displayed impatience, and embarked on a solitary journey. I aspired to soar to great heights and establish my own business involving something linked to creativity. I hadn't contemplated on my purpose; I lacked gratitude, and struggled with self-love. While it's natural to set goals, it's equally vital to savour present moments that often slip by unnoticed. One needs to find inner peace. In the midst of life's chaos, we must spare moments to connect with ourselves. Gradually, a shift in thinking and behaviour unfolds, opening up a new world of understanding. Compared to my previous self, I now possess greater contentment and a profound sense of gratitude for everything in my life. I'm more open-minded, less judgmental, and better equipped to manage my thoughts. Occasionally, I regress into old patterns but remind myself that even that is acceptable. Life presents both roses and thorns, but ultimately, it's our response that shapes our experiences. Cancer taught me to let go of my firm grip on things, enjoy life's moments even in challenging times, and find joy in the small stuff.

Chapter 13
Shedding the Ego

When interacting with cancer patients, I've realized the one common barrier to progress: ego. It's not uncommon for individuals, including myself, to resist change, isolate ourselves, and pursue our own paths when faced with something as daunting as cancer. Accepting that things don't always go according to plan can be incredibly difficult. My marriage had ended, my career faltered, I had to close my store, and now this disease—all combined to deal a devastating blow to my ego.

Cancer compels you to release your grip on the things you cling to tightly. Rigidity is common among cancer patients. As I've learned from holistic practitioners and my own experience, those who are resistant to change often find it challenging to accept their circumstances. In my case, I was incredibly stubborn and resistant to change. Moreover, I habitually pursued the wrong objectives to prove a point. In my journey with cancer, I eventually surrendered, and that's when the healing began.

Chronic diseases originate in the mind with symptoms such as headaches, migraines, aches, pains, and digestive issues preceding physical manifestation of the disease. This is a gradual process, so it's essential to understand the reasons behind these symptoms. Even seemingly minor conditions like high blood pressure can lead to more significant problems. We believe swallowing a pill is the solution to everything, but that's not always the case. Patients with conditions like high blood pressure or diabetes accept these illnesses as normal as they have seen it in their family or received reassurances from doctors. We are conditioned to tolerate these illnesses rather than seek to reverse them. Resistance to change can have long-term consequences, and I've seen many individuals with pre-existing conditions struggle when faced with cancer.

Additionally, their risk of developing other types of cancer can increase if these illnesses are accepted instead of countered proactively. Our bodies are like machines with the organs serving as different components. Just as machines require proper maintenance and lubrication, so do our bodies. Relying solely on medication is a temporary solution, not a long-term fix. While some doctors may insist on lifelong medication, it's not necessarily correct. I've witnessed miraculous recoveries, and many of my patients are now medication-free. Taking medication for conditions like high blood pressure can lead to additional issues impacting the kidneys and potentially necessitating blood thinners, creating a cycle of counteracting effects. If one gets stuck in that vicious circle, sometimes it's just too late to make an impactful change.

My experience with chemotherapy effectively crushed my ego, and I mean it in the best way. It broadened my perspective and shoved me out of my comfort zone, forcing me to take responsibility for my wellbeing. Don't get me wrong; stepping out of your comfort zone and embracing change is intimidating and unsettling. However, when you recognize the potential for a positive outcome, you see the value in taking that leap. This experience compelled me to merge the best aspects of conventional and alternative therapies, adopting a middle path. I received the most effective conventional treatment while enhancing my body's recovery through alternative methods, reducing the duration of my illness.

This experience revealed that I needed to take this path to truly comprehend the anguish cancer patients endure during their treatment and chemotherapy. Often, we fail to deeply analyse the root causes of our suffering or the origins of our diseases. We rarely transition from asking, "Why me?" to declaring, "Try me." This journey has made me a more compassionate person. I've always empathized with others, recognizing that everyone is grappling with their own challenges. Now, before responding with undue harshness, I pause to consider whether such a response is necessary. If there's an alternative way to convey understanding, I opt for that. I firmly believe that if you remain calm, your energy will influence those around you. The energy we project almost instantly impacts others if we remain aware and conscious of this phenomenon. I've encountered many patients, from the rigid and angry to the calm and patient, those living in denial, and more. I've realized I must stay true to myself and my learnings even if convincing everyone is impossible, as not everyone is meant to tread this path. When I don't push too hard and simply remain calm and authentic, patients become more receptive. Sharing my journey and experiences leads them to embrace this healing journey with my guidance.

I wouldn't have experienced this transformation if I had clung to my ego and remained inflexible. It's essential to understand the subtleties of our own egos. With all its challenges, trials, tribulations, and mistakes, my journey was necessary, and I'm grateful for it. It reshaped my life and perspective, positioning me as a catalyst for societal change. It's not an accomplishment that's solely mine; it's a way for a higher power to drive change within me and guide me to a point where I can help others understand their diseases, especially cancer. My cancer experience, challenges, and lessons have equipped me to make a difference in people's lives by instilling hope and positivity.

Chapter 14
Relationship with your Body

Understanding one's body and connecting the dots between past health issues and current conditions is vital to improving wellbeing. Many of these symptoms go unnoticed or are dismissed as minor inconveniences but they can provide valuable insights into underlying health concerns.

My cancer journey forced me to confront my body's needs and recognize the importance of providing proper care, nourishment, and healing. We abuse our bodies through unhealthy dietary choices, excessive medication, accumulated stress, and unprocessed emotional trauma. Eventually, our bodies reach a breaking point, unable to tolerate the burden of toxicity and poor lifestyle choices.

As I reflected on my health history, I began to ask my parents questions about my childhood and the medications I had been prescribed.

This exploration revealed how various factors, including the environment, food, thoughts, and a mother's exposure to toxins during pregnancy can impact a person's health from an early age. I also learned that I was lactose intolerant which shed light on the root causes of my digestive issues, acne, and hormonal imbalances. My cancer diagnosis, specifically Hodgkin's Lymphoma, indicated a compromised lymphatic system that struggled to flush out toxins efficiently, contributing to my frequent illnesses.

Throughout my childhood, I grappled with several health issues that, in hindsight, gave me valuable insights into my overall wellbeing and a deeper understanding of the intricate connection between our physical and emotional wellbeing. In retrospect, these early health experiences were the first whispers from my body, signalling that something was amiss. Regrettably, these symptoms often went unexamined or were dismissed as minor inconveniences.

My parents, for instance, never delved into the underlying causes of my recurring milk-induced vomiting episodes as a child. Instead, they attributed it to my being a fussy eater and resorted to administering various injections to prevent these episodes.

The challenges I faced extended beyond dietary concerns. When my family relocated from bustling Mumbai to the quieter town of Ujjain, I encountered a new set of health issues. The extreme heat in my new environment led to frequent nosebleeds. Additionally, up to the eighth grade, I struggled with constipation. These physical ailments were compounded by emotional turmoil stemming from moving from Mumbai to Ujjain, leaving behind my familiar school, and adapting to an entirely unknown place.

I experienced early puberty, entering this phase in the fifth grade. Another significant health issue I faced during my teenage years was Rosacea acne. I grappled with persistent breakouts on my nose, forehead, and cheeks, leading to redness and inflammation that deeply affected my self-esteem. I tried various treatments, including birth control pills and mild steroids, which provided temporary relief but failed to address the root cause. This condition caused me considerable embarrassment in spite of being popular among my peers.

I frequently fell ill and suffered from various ailments. Even as a child, I suffered from constant sneezing, recurrent colds, and respiratory problems. I was even diagnosed as asthmatic at one point. I was dependent on medication to manage these health issues. I also fell very ill in the tenth grade when I contracted dengue and malaria simultaneously.

Understanding these connections and the body's need for rest, healing, love, and nourishment was pivotal in my journey toward better health and wellbeing. I came to view my body as my first soulmate and true friend, recognizing the significance of treating it with love and respect. This newfound awareness emphasized the importance of early-age self-care to build resilience against the most severe health challenges. I also observed that individuals who maintain a healthy lifestyle from an early age are better equipped to cope with health issues later in life. Conversely, those with unhealthy and laid-back lifestyles face greater challenges when addressing health concerns.

This realization underscored the importance of proactively caring for the body and making informed choices about diet, habits, and overall wellbeing.

Chapter 15
Experiencing Highs and Lows

My first chemotherapy session commenced on February 14, 2017. The treatment plan had six sessions, divided into two parts, each with a 15-day gap, making 12 sessions. Before each chemotherapy session, I had to undergo specific blood tests. In cases where my white blood cell (WBC) count was low, I required additional injections. After completing the first six sessions, a PET scan was scheduled to assess the effectiveness of the drugs.

The memory of that first day is etched in my memory. Before commencing, a bone marrow biopsy was deemed necessary. Despite my reservations, I proceeded without questioning the doctors, maintaining my faith in the medical system. The biopsy procedure was exceedingly painful—it felt like a thousand staples were being inserted into my backbone. The discomfort persisted despite the administering of local anaesthesia. Subsequently, I received two injections in my abdomen to safeguard my ovaries. Following this, I was admitted to the hospital, filled with anticipation and anxiety. Accompanied by my sister and father, I fervently prayed for a positive outcome.

At the hospital, a nurse took my blood pressure and provided a prescription for an extensive list of medications. Seeing this list heightened my anxiety as we waited for the doctor. In the afternoon, the doctor offered some guidance. She cautioned that chemotherapy would be painful, particularly since I couldn't use a chemo port due to the lesions around my chest. I couldn't help but wonder how much more painful it would be compared to the biopsy. I was soon to find out.

When the chemotherapy was administered through a port, the discomfort began. Initially, the sensation was mild, but the intensity rapidly escalated. I experienced a prickly sensation akin to a thousand ants biting me. Despite my cries, I had to endure this pain for thirty minutes. I was thankful when it was finally over, leaving me with a dizzy sensation and vague recollections of my family conversing around me, and visits from my brother-in-law, uncle, and mother offering emotional support. I had no appetite for the hospital meal that followed—mainly tea and soup. I was in severe pain all night, and I couldn't sleep. My back ached and my left hand throbbed. Due to my pronounced weakness, I remained under observation for an entire day.

The next day, I was permitted to go home. However, upon arriving, I began to experience persistent nausea. An unpleasant metallic taste filled my mouth from the medications. I tried to rest but my body ached, and I felt a constant tightening sensation internally. At that moment, I wondered how I would endure the remaining eleven chemotherapy sessions! Despite being prescribed numerous pills by the doctors to mitigate the side effects of the chemotherapy drugs, I struggled with issues such as acidity, oedema, bloating, and continuous nausea. I was advised to consume ice cream and whatever food I could eat as part of my treatment.

A week later, I met with the oncology surgeon to determine whether the placement of a chemo port was feasible. Upon receiving the surgeon's approval, I had to undergo a minor surgical procedure. Despite its minor nature, being wheeled into an operating room on a hospital bed made me feel the most helpless and vulnerable I have ever felt in my life.

Inside the operating room, the surgeon conferred with his colleagues about the tumour and the benefits of placing the port on the left side, as the right side had lesions. There was a brief debate among them, with some suggesting it could be placed on the right despite the proximity to the heart. Ultimately, they made a small incision above my breast and inserted the port on the left side. It felt strange, and I couldn't help but think, "Wow! Now everyone can see my breast!"

Due to the medication, I felt no pain or discomfort but remained groggy. I was then moved to the room where the next round of chemotherapy would commence the following day. I hadn't eaten anything since morning and was famished, but the pain started to set in. I couldn't move my head and felt stiff. After enduring multiple days of this trauma, I was genuinely exhausted. The site of the bone marrow biopsy still hurt, and my hand turned black and blue due to nerve damage. Chemo drugs cause damage and burning in the veins that can take years to heal. Additionally, the site where the port was inserted was also painful. The surgeon came to check on me at night, and I complained about my pain and discomfort. He dismissed it as insignificant, assuring me I would feel better soon.

I was furious. How could he dismiss my pain as nothing? With great effort, I eventually fell asleep with my father sitting by me. In the morning, I thought I could manage alone as I needed to use the restroom. But I blacked out as soon as I stood up. I couldn't even call my dad who was on the phone outside. I tried to cry out but no sound escaped my throat. While it was traumatic at the time, in retrospect, it must have seemed like a scene from a movie where someone is experiencing a heart attack and unable to do anything about it!

The blackout was due to shallow blood pressure because I hadn't eaten anything. I struggled to reach a sitting position and remained there for three minutes. When my dad entered the room, I informed him about the blackout. He made me lie down and gave me water, and I gradually began to feel better. In the afternoon, they initiated the chemotherapy through the port. It was easier than the first time. The following day, I was discharged and returned home to confront new side effects along with some familiar ones—pain, nausea, oedema, weight loss, acne, hot flashes, loss of appetite, and a low WBC (white blood cell) count.

As with all chemo patients, I knew that I would eventually lose my hair, so I had already started researching where to get a wig made. Unfortunately, I had begun this research too late. I had cut my hair short before starting chemotherapy without realizing that wig makers typically use a client's original hair for the wig. Since I didn't have enough hair to make a wig, I met a man specializing in making wigs for the film industry. The encounter was rather peculiar, and my dad and I shared a laugh about it later. You come across so many people who will take advantage of your vulnerability and sickness, so you just have to be mindful about it. Later on, I did get a wig made but he didn't use my hair though.

The studio apartment in Bandra that I had moved into after filing for divorce was too small for my parents and me, especially with my health condition. We decided to look for a larger place—so I spent the time between chemo sessions looking for a suitable home. Eventually, we found a decent 2BHK apartment in Santacruz, conveniently located, and within our budget. The process of moving was physically taxing and emotionally draining. I was weary of constant changes, but I knew it was necessary because my cosy den, which was adequate for me alone, couldn't accommodate all three of us. We completed all the formalities and had to move before the third round of chemotherapy began.

Chapter 16
Importance of Nutrition

I wasn't happy with my diet during the treatment. I was nauseous, acidic, and experienced a profound lack of energy. I felt sad and utterly drained, struggling to rise from the bed every day. Oddly, eating didn't provide the satiation I sought. My body seemed to be crying out for something healthy, recognizing that a change was essential for a speedy recovery. To prevent the cancer from reappearing, I needed a specific dietary regimen. I believed precision nutrition was crucial, a facet often overlooked in mainstream conventional treatments where doctors rarely emphasize its importance. Nevertheless, I was determined to make significant changes in my diet.

My mother introduced me to Dr. Rashmi Menon, a holistic healer who specializes in working with cancer patients. Under her guidance, we adopted a plant-based diet that excluded oil, dairy, gluten, sugar, and animal protein. While it sounded challenging, I was mentally prepared to try it. I had already forsaken most of the items she mentioned, except dairy. Her recommendations resonated with me, so I committed to this change. That marked the end of ghee, butter, milk, buttermilk, chocolates, ice creams, desserts, and bread—all things I had previously cherished. Cancer took me on an educational journey to discern vegan foods from those that aren't, of which there was limited understanding at the time. The divide between vegetarian and vegan products was blurred, making it a trial-and-error phase where I scrutinized all product labels meticulously. When these efforts proved unsuccessful, I resolved not to eat anything from outside and opted to prepare everything at home, allowing me complete control over what I consumed.

My mother even enrolled in cooking classes to grasp the fundamentals of plant-based cooking. Cooking without oil might appear daunting to the average person, but with proper techniques, it becomes manageable and increasingly effortless with practice. Mastering the art of tempering without oil and avoiding utensil damage took some time. To facilitate this, we acquired a set of clay-based cookware for slow cooking. I also incorporated raw organic elements into my diet, including salads, greens, smoothies, fruits, and vegetable juices. I adhered strictly to a rigorous eating schedule. My daily intake featured many vegetables in salad form, including mint leaves, curry leaves, Tulsi, spinach, kale, and more. I introduced berries, dragon fruit, citrus fruits, and other nutrient-rich options to my meals. Consequently, my diet became replete with fibre, phytonutrients, antioxidants, and micronutrients.

There's a common misconception that one should avoid raw food during cancer treatment. In most cases, oncologists advise against it due to concerns about potential infections from unclean fruits and vegetables. However, it's perfectly safe to consume raw foods by being vigilant about using organic produce or thoroughly cleaning them with apple cider vinegar or salt water. For diarrhea or digestive issues, lightly steaming vegetables is recommended while avoiding overcooking or adding excessive oil. Opting for whole fruits over fruit juices is advisable for a well-rounded diet. The challenge of sourcing high-quality organic produce persisted. But my parents undertook this task diligently, visiting farmer's markets or a trusted organic vendor every Sunday.

Consuming calorically dense foods alone makes no sense; the key lies in nutrition-dense foods that promote healing and provide essential energy. Here's an insight into my daily dietary regimen during that period:

Early Morning: I began my day with wheatgrass and Giloy shots (Tinospora Cordoifolia, a herbal plant) to boost immunity.

9:00 AM - A nourishing green smoothie with seasonal fruits like banana and pineapple, along with greens such as spinach, mint, and parsley. I often added soaked chia or pumpkin seeds for an extra nutritional punch.

11:00 AM: Carrot and beetroot juice infused with ginger. If I was still hungry, I added oatmeal.

12:00 Noon: A handful of soaked dry fruits, including almonds, raisins, and walnuts.

1:30 PM: A hearty salad with cucumber, carrots, bell peppers, onions, greens, and tomatoes.

2:00 PM: Wholesome Indian meal, typically with two gluten-free rotis, a sabzi (vegetable dish), and dal (lentils) with green chutney.

4:00 PM: Fruits or makhana (fox nuts) as an afternoon snack.

6:00 PM: Vegetable soup

7:00 PM: One-pot meal, such as khichdi.

Knowing which supplements to take during cancer treatment is crucial, as some may potentially interfere with your ongoing medical regimen. While this area can be quite contentious, consulting with an integrated doctor or a cancer specialist can provide clarity. It became apparent that medication and the dietary shift were taking a toll on my gut health. I experienced frequent, loud burping after meals, indicating prolonged digestion times. This persisted until I took proactive steps to restore my gut health following chemotherapy. I introduced some supplements into my routine, including mushroom tea, curcumin, ashwagandha, multivitamins, Vitamin D, and Vitamin B12. Additionally, I explored homeopathic remedies to bolster my immunity, recognizing it as a holistic approach in its own right.

Incorporating meditation and visualization techniques played a significant role in my journey, fostering a positive outlook. Unwavering belief is vital to approaching cancer holistically. When we consult medical professionals, we trust them blindly, following their guidance without question. I'm not challenging the remarkable advances made by the medical community, but it's worth noting that holistic practices have thrived for centuries in various cultures, including indigenous tribes known for their longevity and robust health. Take, for example, the Hunza tribe residing in Pakistan's northern mountainous region, reputed to live up to 120 years. Many scientists have studied them, attributing their longevity to factors like an anti-inflammatory diet, a sense of purpose, strong social and spiritual connections, and happiness. Globally, Blue Zones are regions where people enjoy extended, healthy lives. These communities share characteristics such as a sense of fulfillment, close interactions, love, adherence to a healthy diet, and regular exercise to maintain overall wellbeing.

My regimen of wholesome nutrition, meditation, and yoga brought about a remarkable transformation within me. It was a new experience where I nourished my body and gained insights on how it responded to wholesome meals. The difference between how I felt now, following a balanced diet, and my previous state was palpable. This newfound vitality encouraged me to make more beneficial choices. The first decision was to discontinue taking hormone injections. Astonishingly, my acne began to recede almost immediately.

Over time, I furthered my holistic living by reconsidering my personal care products. I phased out conventional shampoos, soaps, and perfumes and replaced my utensils with clay alternatives. Recognizing the potential harm of carcinogenic chemicals, I swapped household items like Harpic, utensil cleaners, floor mop liquids, and hand wash for natural alternatives like raakh, reminiscent of yesteryear practices. This time served as an eye-opener for discovering the abundance of harmful products that escape our attention and awareness, posing risks to us and the environment.

My journey towards healing also encompassed environmental adjustments. I consciously reduced my mobile phone usage, refraining from keeping it near me at night due to concerns about radiation's potential link to cancer. My choice of attire evolved as well, as I now favoured cotton and loose-fitting clothing to allow my skin to breathe freely. I started consuming boiled water as a precaution against infections, later trying ozone water after learning about its potential advantages.

Ozone therapy emerged as an ally in my quest for wellness, reducing inflammation, alleviating oxidative stress, and enhancing cellular functions. This was grounded in the understanding that ozone, with its three oxygen atoms, represents an active form of this vital element. Dr. Otto Warburg's research in 2019 emphasized the crucial role of oxygen in cellular health, leading to the growing emphasis on hyperbaric oxygen therapy. It was eye-opening to realize that the declining oxygen levels in our atmosphere, down by 30 percent, could contribute to conditions like cancer and respiratory disorders.

https://www.sciencenews.org/article/medicine-nobel-2019-discovery-how-cells-sense-oxygen-cancer-wins

The way my life transformed was nothing short of revolutionary. I initiated these dietary and lifestyle changes before my third session of chemotherapy, and it just so happened that this time, after chemo, I experienced minimal nausea. Incorporating lemon water during the treatment played a role in this shift. My diet had become more alkaline, and this change made all the difference. I now understood acidic and alkaline foods and witnessed tangible improvements in my bloating, energy levels, and appetite. Remarkably, I even resumed work, taking up a bridal trousseau order. My clients displayed tremendous kindness by coming to me so that I could work with them.

One of the most distressing aspects of chemotherapy is hair loss, something I thought I was prepared for, but found heart-wrenching when it actually occurred. The prospect of losing my thick, beautiful, and long hair was one of my main worries when I received my cancer diagnosis. It's funny how the human mind goes to the superficial aspect of beauty even when life is at risk.

It was a deeply emotional journey to watch my hair fall away. Then, one day, I reached a breaking point and decided I couldn't bear it any longer. I told my father I wanted to shave my head and have a wig made. Sitting in the barber's chair, I reminded myself that nothing in life is permanent. Gazing into the mirror, I mentally prepared myself not to overthink. "Just let it go, Shruti, you'll get better," I whispered, silently wishing for straighter hair.

I couldn't bring myself to watch as the barber shaved my head and I avoided looking down to witness my beloved tresses falling. When it was over, I examined my reflection and realized I didn't look as bad as I feared. Many of my friends even thought I resembled Persis Khambatta, the model and actress who shaved her head for a Hollywood movie. Although I acquired various accessories and hats to conceal my baldness, the absence of hair was a unique and refreshing sensation. There was no more need for shampooing or other hair products, and I felt lighter in many ways. Wearing a wig was an amusing experience, making me feel like an entirely different person.

At that time, I had to start the process of obtaining an Aadhar card, which proved overwhelming as it needed to be linked to my bank and other entities. I had to enlist the help of an agent to navigate the bureaucracy. The effort put a dent in my enthusiasm, and I found that there were moments when I struggled to muster the strength to feel positive. During these times, questions about the purpose behind it all arose. Contemplating these matters left me feeling drained and weak. The internal struggles of a cancer patient are known only to them; nobody else truly understands.

Sometimes, I yearned to step outside without my wig, but my confidence didn't always align with that desire. However, this experience taught me a profound lesson: letting go of artificial beauty notions. True beauty should not be assessed solely based on outward appearance but on what lies within. Thankfully, I recognized that this situation was not permanent, an epiphany I now share with my clients, especially the women. I understand the emotional impact of losing one's hair, but I reassure them that it's okay to surrender. After all, it's just hair and 99 percent of the time, it grows back. As for me, my hair is now even better in terms of quality and texture. Of course, it's still not perfectly straight, but who cares?!

Chapter 17
Rejoicing in the Victory

As the chemotherapy continued, I began to notice a significant change in my condition. The tumours were gradually melting away—I could no longer feel their presence as distinctly. My neck's mobility also improved gradually. One night, just before my fourth chemotherapy session, while meditating, I had a powerful intuition that the cancer was gone and that I was healed. This intuition was so powerful that I felt compelled to take immediate action by consulting with my doctors. My CRP levels were within the normal range, but I knew that definitive confirmation would come only from a PET scan. A scan was scheduled halfway through the treatment, after six rounds of chemotherapy. Of course, undergoing a PET scan meant exposing myself to radiation, which could be harmful, but I was persistent in my conviction. While more advanced tests are available, such as liquid biopsies that analyse blood samples to determine the extent of cancer present, I needed to validate my intuition. Throughout the process, I prayed fervently, as I always did during PET scans, but this time, I was brimming with confidence about the results.

When I presented the reports to my doctor, I saw joy in her eyes. "There's no cancer in your body. It has stopped metastasizing."

The news was like music to my ears. I eagerly inquired if this meant I could stop the chemotherapy, but she explained that there was a prescribed protocol to follow. They couldn't stop the treatment in case any minuscule cancer cells still lingered. I felt a twinge of disappointment at having to continue with chemotherapy every fifteen days. Upon returning home, I decided to celebrate this incredible milestone with my parents. I couldn't be more grateful to them; they had been unwavering pillars of support throughout my journey. They were by my side every single day. My dad sat through all my chemotherapy sessions while my mom was a constant source of motivation, meticulously monitoring my nutrition and ensuring I had the best possible food.

Having someone to care for you while dealing with cancer is incredibly important. There are countless emotions to grapple with along the way. Even though my journey wasn't over, and more chemotherapy sessions lay ahead, my relationship with my parents underwent a profound transformation. I grew closer to them, openly discussing and resolving any lingering resentments. I felt an overwhelming sense of ease and peace in our connection. It's crucial to communicate openly about your thoughts and feelings.

Since I had already conquered my fear with the belief that the cancer was gone, I faced the remaining chemotherapy sessions with a fearless attitude. Chemotherapy sessions five through eight went smoothly. I was able to work and even venture out occasionally. It was a delightful surprise when my grandmother and cousins visited me. My mom prepared gluten-free pav bhaji and baked a cake for the occasion, making it extra special. However, by the end of the day, I was thoroughly exhausted. Despite my significant improvements, my body still required ample rest, mostly due to the effects of chemotherapy.

The final stretch of chemotherapy was undoubtedly the most challenging, as my body's immunity had been severely compromised by this point. After one of the chemo sessions, I developed a fever of 101 degrees. Alarmed, we rushed to the hospital, and the doctors advised us not to take any risks. Miraculously, my fever disappeared as soon as I was admitted, but I had to continue with the intravenous treatments and medication. I realized I should have waited patiently as the body often raises its temperature to combat viruses and germs. Later, I learned that drugs like Paracetamol can affect the gut, and fever is the body's natural defence. Ideally, one should allow the body to deal with it, rest, consume light meals, and get plenty of sleep. Those two days in the hospital were an unnecessary expense but a valuable learning experience that I use today as a Cancer Coach.

Following this hospitalization, I began seeking treatment at a private clinic in Bandra called Empire. It was a refreshing change from the hospital environment. Very few patients frequented this clinic, and I was able to go home on the same day after a chemo session. I appealed to my doctor that I couldn't take it any more, but stopping the treatment was not an option. Due to the cessation of my periods, I was battling mouth sores, weight loss, extreme sensitivity in my teeth, a heightened sense of smell, and night sweats. But I still had a journey ahead of me, and I was counting down the days till this ordeal ended.

I was having a difficult time with my treatment when I received the news that one of my cousins had been diagnosed with colon cancer. It served as a stark reminder that cancer can affect anyone and that life is incredibly fragile. He, too, adopted significant lifestyle changes and underwent a major surgery. Now, all I could think about was completing my chemotherapy and moving forward. However, questions loomed about life after chemo. How would I rebuild my life? Where would I live it?

Around the time of my tenth chemo session, my dad met with an accident on the road, resulting in significant injuries. He developed a high fever and was diagnosed with a stomach infection. My mom had to juggle responsibilities, caring for two unwell family members. I asked everyone to be by my side when the twelfth and final chemo session arrived. The relief was palpable. We spoke to the doctor who advised specific blood tests and a PET scan after fifteen days, followed by a meeting with her.

Usually, chemo medications would make me groggy, and I would be half-asleep for the rest of the day. However, I recall going home the night after my last chemo and savouring my mom's homemade vegan ice cream before drifting off to sleep. I woke up the next day with a sigh of relief. Now, I had to confront and overcome the cumulative side effects of all those chemotherapy sessions, including:

1. Repairing my gut - Chemo destroys the mucosal lining as it houses the fastest growing cells. That's why people experience loose stools or constipation as we lose good bacteria and that causes belching and acidity. I was belching and had indigestion.

2. Battling fatigue - Because of low iron and low haemoglobin, one gets easily tired. Sometimes the heart can get affected. I had to work on my energy levels.

3. Rebuilding my immunity - The WBC count falls, and it takes time to build it back up as it gets destroyed by chemo drugs that cannot differentiate between good and bad cells.

4. Dealing with hair loss - I lost all my hair and I was so concerned about how it would grow back. It all depends on the hormones and nutrition.

5. Addressing hormonal health - My periods had stopped and I didn't know whether they would start again. I had to cleanse and balance my hormones. I had hot flashes in the night, and I was always estrogen dominant. I experienced pain in my breasts because of fibrosis.

6. Building muscle and strength - I wished I knew this then, but weight training helps in building muscles. I had lost a lot of muscle mass and had to build that with a good intake of proteins and amino acids.

7. Improving my sleep - My sleep was haphazard as I was always a light sleeper. So I had to work on improving it.

8. Managing stress - Being aware of my stress triggers and doing something about it. Not living in denial but really accepting and developing strategies to overcome it were things I had to learn.

9. Addressing mouth sores and gum health - Improving gum health was so important. As a side effect of chemo, the body heats up. The pitta (fire) rises and causes damage so I had to handle it with Vitamin B, aloe vera, and good nutrition.

10. Handling lymphedema - I experienced this for a long time because of poor circulation. I had to up my mineral levels, especially magnesium.

In the days that followed, my diet mainly consisted of semi-solid foods because my gums were too weak to handle anything else. Ulcers in my throat made it difficult to swallow, but I told myself, "This, too, shall pass." I was determined to get better, and I found that affirmations were incredibly powerful; it truly was a case of mind over matter.

To my readers, I want to emphasize that good health can indeed be manifested. It's all about consistency and persistence. Often, we seek instant gratification and quick results, but real progress takes time. I was prepared for the journey ahead, knowing that my gut would take more than two years to repair, my hair would need almost a year to grow back, and the status of my hormones was uncertain. Building muscle and strength would take patience, just like my other challenges. All I needed was a comprehensive health strategy and a plan for each day, week, and year.

Chapter 18
A Medical Dilemma

My chemotherapy concluded in August, and my parents had to return to the United States to reapply for my green card. It had been rejected by the US embassy due to a regrettable decision I had made—changing my surname after marriage.

My parents didn't want me to remain in Mumbai until my immigration situation was resolved, so I decided to relocate to Jaipur. I had relatives there, it was a tier 2 city, and I was yearning for a change from the city life that had caused me so much stress. I felt the urgent need to escape and not encounter the same people, or reside in the same locality.

In the second week of August, I underwent another round of scans, fully expecting them to come back clear. However, when I visited my doctor, I was shocked to head that I needed radiation therapy. I couldn't comprehend why I was being advised to undergo radiation when my reports showed no signs of cancer. The doctor explained that it was a preventive measure to reduce the risk of a relapse, especially since the tumour in my neck still needed addressing. I remained puzzled because I firmly believed that I was cancer-free. The situation caught me off guard.

I consulted a radiologist with all my reports, seeking a more detailed explanation of how radiation therapy worked. Because the tumour was on my neck, this treatment was deemed necessary to prevent its return. Despite his explanations, doubts crept into my mind, and I questioned my choices again. Memories of my past decisions resurfaced, and I couldn't help but wonder if I had made a mistake pursuing natural therapies.

My doctor pointed out, "You've already taken a risk once. Why take another one?"

I sat in a cab with my mom, both of us feeling utterly confused about what to do next. I had already decided to leave Mumbai, and the prospect of radiation was terrifying, especially considering the potential risk of developing thyroid problems later on. I wanted to step back, think things over, and seek a second opinion, which I obtained from my homeopathic doctor. He advised against radiation, emphasizing the need to examine my reports closely and weigh the logic. As a holistic doctor, his perspective resonated with my desire to trust my intuition and make an informed choice.

Now, as a healer myself, I understand the dilemmas that many of my patients face when deciding whether to undergo artificial hormonal therapy (taking Tamoxifen and Olaparib) or radiation, despite clear scan results. The choice depends on the type of cancer, its stage, the patient's age, and, most significantly, their confidence in their chosen path. I told myself, "Let me take this chance and give myself another six months. I will apply everything I've learned and work towards healing myself. I'll monitor my progress, strengthen my immunity, and then assess whether radiation is still necessary." Given my impending move, I informed my doctor that I would undergo radiation therapy in Jaipur to avoid further arguments.

Doctors practicing allopathy believe that no other techniques have an impact on cancer. Numerous clinical experiments have demonstrated the power of the placebo effect where patients are given a sugar pill instead of actual medication. They are informed that it's medicine, and remarkably, they begin to feel better. This highlights the mind's capacity to be deceived and how an individual's belief system can influence their wellbeing. I recognized that I needed to apply these same principles to my own healing journey. I had to embrace a placebo-effect mentality, convincing my mind that I was cancer-free and living a healthy life in the desired end state, a fundamental principle of manifestation.

Chapter 19

Taking Small Steps

Now that chemotherapy was complete, I embarked on a journey of self-recovery with my health as my top priority. It was a challenging decision for someone like me, an inherently anxious individual who thrived on juggling multiple tasks simultaneously. However, I recognized the need to slow down and give my body the required attention. Even if it meant temporarily setting aside my career and the activities I loved, I understood that healing had to come first.

I created a post-chemo recovery road map around several crucial steps:

1. Cleansing my Gut: Chemotherapy leaves behind dead cells and debris in the gut, particularly affecting the lymphatic system. I focused on an extended anti-inflammatory diet, rich in gut-healing foods and incorporated coffee enemas three times a week.

2. Hormone Balancing: Ever since my menstrual cycle had halted, I experienced breast fibrosis, hot flashes, and erratic sleep. Uncertain whether my periods would ever return,I introduced the external application of castor oil packs on my uterus twice a week not only benefited the liver, but also addressed fibroids and cleansed the uterus.

3. Exercise and Yoga: Regular walks, restorative yoga sessions, and pranayama were non-negotiable in my daily routine. These practices played a vital role in my recovery.

4. Regulating Sleep: I adopted specific poses, such as Balasana, chanted Om, and practiced Bhramari Pranayama to improve my sleep quality. Frequent afternoon naps helped manage my fatigue.

5. Building Strength: Prioritizing a protein-rich diet supplemented with amino acids and plant-based protein boosters aided in rebuilding my strength.

6. Boosting Immunity: I incorporated herbs like curcumin and ashwagandha into my diet to enhance my immune system.

7. Meditation for Mental Peace: Despite maintaining a positive outlook, there was an underlying fear of cancer returning. Overcoming this fear required consistent meditation and staying grounded in the present moment.

I was committed to my yoga practice which added so much value to my life by calming my mind while healing my body. I never missed a session; I even kept a workout journal to help me maintain discipline and consistency. Over the course of a year, I exercised approximately 200 out of 365 days. I firmly believe that consistency and discipline are essential to good health. It was hard initially, but I persisted. I was excited about what was coming up next for me as I could feel that something significant was around the corner. For now, I focused on building myself and shut out everything else.

Never underestimate the power of food and nutrition. People dismiss the impact of their dietary choices because they are conditioned to believe that what they consider 'healthy' aligns with what's genuinely beneficial for their bodies and souls. Changing eating patterns can be difficult, especially when emotions and unconscious habits are intertwined. This revelation was transformative for me in altering my food habits and other aspects, from choosing what to wear to consciously avoiding products that harm the environment or animals. I gave up all products that harmed the environment or animals, like leather products and silk. It felt like a natural transition now that I was following a plant-based diet, and it came from within. As the choices in my daily life changed, the way I reacted to things changed, as did the way I wanted to lead my life.

Around six months into my recovery, I attended a lecture by Sadhguru in Jaipur. While I had no expectations regarding my menstrual cycle, something prompted me to carry a sanitary napkin. During the meditation session, I suddenly felt overwhelmed and started crying, sensing a surge of energy within me. To my surprise, I had started my period and it stained my clothes.

Yet, I was elated because it signified the reactivation of my ovaries and it felt like confirmation that I was on the right path to recovery.

Chapter 20
A Pivotal Stage

My application for the US green card was rejected once more. I wasn't disheartened but my mother was distraught as she had to return to the US. I decided to remain in Jaipur where I had the support of my aunt, uncle, cousins, and nephews. Their care and presence were comforting, but the uncertainty of my future still loomed. Would I be able to maintain my health routine and dietary discipline without my mother by my side? The responsibility now fell squarely on my shoulders, and I had to stay on track.

Once I settled into a routine in Jaipur, I contemplated the next steps for my career. I felt a strong desire to give back to society, but how to do that in the fashion industry? It occurred to me I could make a difference in sustainable fashion. I enrolled in an online fashion course from CSF, London, a prestigious institution, which expanded my knowledge and provided fresh insights. Very few brands practiced sustainability then, so I saw the potential in doing so, particularly in Jaipur, a fashion hub. I began networking, learning about natural and organic fabrics and dyes, and eventually launched my brand, EHCORE (eco to the core). I initiated collaborations with rural women, empowering them through employment. Witnessing the daughter of one of these women go to college thanks to her mother's earnings from our brand filled me with immense satisfaction.

Soon, I embarked on my first solo trip to Pondicherry and Auroville. A friend initially accompanied me to Auroville, but I extended my stay by four additional days. It was a liberating experience as I made decisions regarding activities, destinations, and meals. I interacted with strangers, formed friendships, and relished my own company. This newfound independence was a revelation for me. Cancer patients often grapple with diminished confidence, and certain life events had left me feeling lonely, particularly my mother's return to the US. I realized that if I needed to embrace independence and tackle things on my own, why not start with solo travel? Auroville offered the perfect blend of tranquillity, serenity, and healthy lifestyle options. I also indulged in rejuvenating therapies like shiatsu (a combination of kneading, pressing, tapping and stretching techniques that reduce tension and re-energise the body).

Simultaneously, I started mingling in different communities in Jaipur to connect with like-minded individuals. At one of these meetups where I shared my cancer journey, I had the privilege of meeting NKC Sir from Jaipur Rugs. Unbeknownst to me, he was a humble and influential figure. After I had recounted my cancer journey, he took my contact information and later invited me to meet him. During our meeting, he suggested I visit his organization's premises and explore the villages where the artisans crafted rugs. I was captivated by his story and mission. He then asked me to give a lecture about my journey at his corporate office. This was a significant step for me, as I was quite shy. The response from the audience left me astonished and humbled as I witnessed the impact of sharing my story.

Sometimes, we forget to applaud ourselves but this experience encouraged me to do just that. I was also invited for lunch during which NKC Sir expressed his fascination with a single sentence I had mentioned about letting go. He shared his desire to work on his health and extended an invitation to me to join Jaipur Rugs. I was surprised and intrigued; I had never worked in a corporate setting. Nevertheless, I agreed without overthinking it. This marked my initial foray into health coaching while I was still working on my own sustainable fashion label. To be working on two things I loved made me so grateful to the universe.

Gradually I felt myself drawn more and more towards health coaching. Motivating and helping people was so rewarding. Even my fashion brand was helping women who were living alone and struggling. I was able to sponsor a girl's college fees which felt amazing. One coach I spoke to presented me with a difficult question—if I had to choose one thing, fashion or coaching, what would it be? I choose to be a full-fledged health coach. During Covid, it so happened that I had to let go of my fashion label and begin working full-time as a coach, based on my life-experiences rather than formal qualifications. From this point onwards, my confidence grew and I realized that this was my calling. I wanted to delve deeper into healing the human mind and body, and I had an open invitation to expand my knowledge and skills in this field.

Finding passion

When we encounter adversity, we often label it as a negative event without fully comprehending the potential lessons or opportunities it might hold. Thinking positively may seem impossible at that time, but if we can understand its purpose, these challenges can transform into remarkable experiences. In hindsight, I've come to view cancer as a guiding force in my life, steering me toward positive changes I would never have contemplated otherwise. It spurred transformation in my habits, lifestyle, and mindset, even leading me to write this book. Conquering cancer has been profoundly humbling, and it has endowed me with the strength to face minor troubles with resilience. Whenever life's challenges arise now, I simply remind myself of what I have already overcome, and then my troubles don't seem insurmountable anymore.

I always remember the powerful intuition I experienced during my meditation practice after the fourth chemotherapy session. I felt a calling to do something meaningful for people battling cancer. It was a profound urge to channel the knowledge I had acquired into a force for good. I didn't fully understand the significance of this feeling at the time, but I accepted the idea and asked the universe to guide me. The opportunity to fulfil this calling presented itself when I began working as a health coach in Jaipur. This role granted me invaluable insights into people's psychology and eating habits. Regardless of social strata, I discovered that everyone faced health-related challenges, each with unique issues. Through consultations with over a hundred individuals, I diligently recorded their concerns and helped them make better lifestyle choices.

In collaboration with Jaipur Rugs, we initiated a holistic department, introducing mindfulness and yoga sessions and implementing significant changes in the workplace cafeteria. We took steps to reduce plastic waste by replacing plastic bottles with steel ones. NKC Sir wholeheartedly supported these initiatives. I began organizing workshops and vegan meetups, which brought me immense joy. I also began giving talks and working alongside organizations like Sharan run by Dr. Nandita Shah, a pioneer in holistic healing without using medicine, who was one of the first to start the vegan movement in India.

Positively impacting people's lives enriched me in ways I never imagined. I blossomed in every sense; my hair grew back and my periods resumed their regular cycle. Slowly but surely, I regained physical strength, although I was skinnier than before. I became acutely aware of crucial aspects that cancer survivors should remember. I learned from numerous practitioners that one must exercise caution with their lifestyle choices, especially during the three years following treatment. Official remission is declared only after five years. When I observe cancer relapses in patients, it is primarily because they return to their usual lifestyles after completing the treatment, which is a critical mistake. Conventional treatments don't guarantee that cancer won't return; addressing the root cause is the key. I encourage all cancer survivors to transform their lifestyles and always maintain faith, for miracles occur every day.

One of the most profound realizations stemming from my battle with cancer was recognizing that I had been missing a deep sense of purpose in my life. When one is determined to heal and contribute positively, even the cloudiest days can't dull their light. Living in depression and unfulfillment can adversely affect genes and immunity. These lead to elevated cortisol levels, which may contribute to cancer, as confirmed by nearly 99% of the cancer patients I conversed with.

When I visited my doctor a year later, my enthusiasm and transformation left her so impressed, that she sought my advice on weight loss. It was so sweet of her to ask me—she even pushed me to start a motivational channel. I remained vigilant about routine tests and check-ups for two years. The port required regular flushing in case of cancer recurrence, serving as a constant reminder to stay cautious. The tumour marks on my neck that I had initially found so unsightly were now symbols of bravery and resilience, and I no longer cared about concealing them. My sole focus was fortifying my immunity to ensure that the cancer never returned.

I adopted various measures to protect myself from radiation, a pervasive threat in today's tech-driven world. Whether it was volcanic ash or

Shungite crystals, I employed various remedies to absorb radiation. I abstained from using synthetic perfumes and chemical skincare products, prioritized regular detoxification, and maintained essential vitamin and mineral levels, including vitamin D, B12, magnesium, and selenium. I also rotated my supplements and consciously avoided falling into self-pity or depression, redirecting my energy toward activities that brought me joy.

Every cancer patient embarks on their unique journey. Mine led me to become a healer of sorts. My tone of voice transformed, exuding a sense of calm that resonated with people. I created a safe space free from judgment where individuals felt comfortable opening up to me and sharing their stories. Many have shed tears and unburdened their hearts to me, revealing the depths of their pain. I am deeply grateful to them, as they taught me invaluable lessons on how to approach people with compassion and provide them with a sense of security and a listening ear. Having experienced unkindness from some individuals, I realized that irrespective of the trials people endure, it costs nothing to be kind to them even if they are rude.

As a coach, I've had the privilege of counselling couples, parents and men and women who carry deep traumas, without a formal degree or training. I have made a meaningful difference in their lives. This experience instilled in me a profound sense of confidence in my calling. I yearned to learn more and contribute to creating a world free from disease and suffering.

All diseases originate in the mind and then manifest in the body; a fundamental truth. I once visualized a dagger in my back during a challenging period with my ex-husband, and that thought manifested into reality. It was my soul's way of crying out, demanding attention, care, and self-love. I changed careers in my late thirties, taking a leap of faith in myself and my ability to transform lives just as I had transformed my own. I aimed to set an example and help others do the same, and I was fortunate that people trusted me with their health and challenges.

Opportunities

At Jaipur Rugs, I worked closely with many individuals and that helped me discover the intricate connections between the mind and the body. I witnessed firsthand how dietary changes can improve overall wellbeing. Productivity increased and a newfound positivity emerged. It's often said that one healthy person can positively impact the lives of four others, and I experienced this phenomenon. I gained invaluable experience in holistically assisting people with a wide array of health issues, including diabetes, thyroid problems, hypertension, anxiety, obesity, and autoimmune conditions.

By focusing on mindfulness, gratitude, and meditation, people heal faster. I encountered young men who opened up about their struggles with suicidal thoughts and unhappiness. Their reports indicated deficiencies in essential nutrients, such as Vitamin D, and other nutritional gaps. By addressing the nutritional deficiencies, adjusting thought patterns, and altering lifestyle choices, they transformed into happier and more fulfilled human beings. One gentleman shared how he had regained his happiness, pursued his passions, and formed a community of like-minded individuals in his area. Witnessing these transformations was deeply rewarding and validating.

My story was touching people in meaningful ways. I organized vegan potlucks and was delighted to see a diverse group of people attending, sharing their journeys, and savouring healthy food with joy. Most were pleasantly surprised by the delicious and nutritious meals. My seminars, talks, and workshops allowed me to connect with people, listen to their stories and challenges, and gain new perspectives. Gradually, I developed confidence in public speaking and communicating through various media.

The year 2020 brought unprecedented challenges as the COVID-19 pandemic swept across the globe. People suddenly realized the fragility of life and the importance of health. Despite the grimness of the situation, it provided me the opportunity to conduct online workshops and create a virtual community. I also facilitated fasting for nearly a hundred individuals online through social media and WhatsApp and found it to be a fulfilling experience.

It was the perfect time to acquire new knowledge, so I enrolled in some courses to expand my horizons. At this time, I also began working with cancer patients, particularly those who had experienced relapses. I felt a deep empathy for them, knowing their struggles intimately. I knew that shifting their mindsets was a challenging yet achievable goal, The pandemic presented the chance to relocate to Goa, India, seeking more freedom, fresh air, and a closer connection to nature. My time there afforded me the space to contemplate my next steps and continue on my path of healing and transformation.

Taking a leap of faith

I felt a strong calling to create a platform to provide cancer patients with comprehensive, well-researched, evidence-based, and result-oriented protocols whether they pursue conventional treatments or holistic protocols. This platform would encompass supplements, products, books, therapists, and yoga teachers, all easily accessible online, allowing individuals to navigate their healing journey at their own pace and in the comfort of their own space. This vision stemmed from the challenges I faced when sifting through various materials to determine what would truly benefit my body in the fight against cancer. My desire was to curate a tangible resource and share it with the world.

However, I was unsure whether to establish a proprietorship firm or involve others in my endeavour. The entrepreneurial journey can be likened to a roller coaster ride, and I had already weathered its toll. The most crucial aspect was to make a difference in people's lives by sharing my journey and knowledge with the world. I began laying out plans for addressing different diseases and consulted integrated doctors and naturopaths who generously shared their insights and encouraged me to move forward. My goal was to provide cancer patients and those with chronic diseases access to information about the best supplements, products, and guidance on sourcing, usage, and energy protection.

As time passed, I realized the necessity of building a team to bring this vision to life. In 2021, I crossed paths with my partner who played a pivotal role in developing the brand strategy and website, ultimately leading to the birth of Awaana Health. Our journey to reach our current point was filled with its fair share of challenges and triumphs. Convincing doctors and healers to come on board was an uphill battle, and it was a reminder that success often conceals the hard work that goes on behind the scenes.

I believe I've only just begun, and now, I serve a global clientele. Collaborating with individuals from different nationalities has expanded my perspective on merging Eastern and Western philosophies to create holistic modules aimed at helping more and more people. The fundamental idea behind Awaana Health is to offer a 360-degree approach to health and wellbeing. This approach encompasses nutrition, holistic therapies, mental health support, and empowerment. It provides individuals, especially cancer patients, with a one-stop resource where they can access everything they need during a challenging and confusing time, ultimately empowering them to take control of their health and wellbeing.

In November 2021, I got my green card and decided to move to the USA to be with my parents as they needed my support. My dad's health was suffering as a side effect of taking BP medication for 30 plus years. As he suffered from chronic kidney disorder, I was required to help him with his health. It was a difficult move for me as I had to make some major decisions with my team about being in the USA and working odd hours, but I was determined to make it work. I have had many ups and downs during this journey but when you are determined to make a difference in people's lives, doors open. I've started working more internationally, and I've found that people are more open to holistic practices, though most initiatives come from India.

I have also finally got my Energy Psychology certificate and completed an FLNA course in functional medicine. I am now doing more and more energy work—helping people unblock their energy and get rid of traumas and past burdens. I try to help them make the self-realization journey happy and easy so that people take full responsibility for their own mental health.

Working one on one with people, it is fascinating to observe how and where the body stores trauma and releases it. I have developed my own flows of yoga and movement therapy. I have also built a community that meets once a week and talks about limitations, resistances, and blockages. We motivate each other—I find this so useful, especially for cancer patients. I want it to grow exponentially, and have faith that it will.

My next project is to develop a recipe book for cancer patients, and I am also excited to be working on a digital course that will be released in different languages. I plan to continue serving people and come up with more and more books. This is just the beginning for me! My mission is to empower individuals facing a cancer diagnosis, encouraging them to explore a comprehensive approach that combines conventional treatments with holistic methodologies. I believe that, in addition to the standard medical path, embracing a holistic perspective can contribute positively to their overall wellbeing and journey toward healing

Cancer has 'CAN' in it, symbolizing the strength within. Everyone can overcome it with resilience and determination.

In Search of the Right Approach

I have met many pathbreaking doctors, healers and guides on my journey and I am deeply grateful to all of them. Let me take you through how their expertise and mindset helped me make the right choices.

Dr Milli Arpan Shah - BHMS (BOM), MS (Counselling and Psychotherapy), President of Ozone Forum, India, has this to say:

"My journey in ozone therapy started way back in 2005 when I was introduced to it by one of my friends. It was an excellent complementary and supportive alternative therapy that originated in Germany, where a lot of scientific data has been observed and analysed. The main feature of ozone-based therapy is treating the root cause and improving the patient holistically. When we treat patients with ozone therapy, the treatment is from inside to out, and that's how it gives beautiful results for chronic, degenerative diseases.

Regarding cancer—from 2006 to 2007, I worked with a radiologist in the radiation department of Lady Ratan Tata Medical Centre, where we experimented with ozone therapy to help radiation patients improve their outcomes. Many patients cannot tolerate the side effects of radiation, thus they drop out; therefore, the treatment rate or success is limited. When we did ozone therapy for 83 radiation patients, their treatment outcomes were very good. They did not have any metastasis for nine months to a year and did not have any complications from radiation. At the same time, the tumour markers were controlled. This paper was published, and since then, we have been practicing ozone therapy with cancer patients as an integrator in oncology.

My fundamentals in using ozone therapy are based on the 3P model: Psychology, Physiology and Pathophysiology. We talk to the patient and help them overcome their psychological burden. I firmly believe that all cancer is metaphysical; it starts at the emotional level and manifests at the physical level. So, helping the psychology of the patient is very important. Coming to physiology, ozone therapy rectifies the oxygenation in the body. All cancer patients have hypoxic shock—through ozone therapy we convert that hypoxic shock to normoxic, improving their circulation. Regarding pathophysiology, ozone's bio-oxidative work helps reduce oxidative stress caused by cancer.

In my opinion, looking at alternative therapies for cancer is vital. You should look at why it happened, what was the trigger, what carcinogenic factors are present in the body, and what important causative factors should be removed. And it cannot be done only by chemo and radiation; one must look holistically. First, at food, then, the mind, third, the Circadian rhythm. Whenever a cancer patient undergoes treatment, they must address all the other parameters through lifestyle modification, food modification, nutrition improvement, and working on psychology. So, everything is necessary; holistic treatment and integration are the future. I think it's better to start with oncology because many people don't die from cancer; they die from treatment complications. So, I strongly prefer that all cancer patients take supportive, integrated medical help.

When Shruti came to us for treatment, I saw that she was slightly depressed. In the starting phase, she was in denial, questioning why this had happened to her. I remember talking with her for hours; she had come with her mother who was also positively influenced by natural living. Getting Shruti to accept that this would help her was easy. We tried ozone therapy and Vitamin C. The first dietary changes we suggested for her were to reduce carbs and sugar and go holistic in her eating. She was very positively motivated to look after herself. When she needed chemotherapy, I told her, "Yes, you should always look at the whole picture, so if chemo fits the jigsaw puzzle of your healing, you should do it." My relationship with Shruti was supportive and complementary. I was always there if she had any queries, and it was good that she followed all my advice properly. Today, when she is writing this book, I'm so amazed and happy for her and how she has evolved during these years. Congratulations to you, Shruti, for this.

The major drawback of conventional cancer treatment is that they just treat the upper layer—like the tip of an iceberg. They don't look below the iceberg to see what caused it. For cancer, you need to treat the root-level causes. So, conventional treatment in acute conditions is required and useful, but at the same time, holistic treatment advice is always good."

***

Dr Raj Merchant – MD. Naturopathy

"I got into the field of Naturopathy because of my grandmother who was heavily diabetic. Her foot was full of pus and maggots and she was advised to get her leg amputated from above the knee. I met a guruji called Mukherjee Babu who helped me to save her leg. She lived for another ten years with no need for amputation. She was cured entirely with herbs.

I felt like learning this, so in the year 1967, I went to stay with him in the jungle for an education on plants and leaves. He didn't live in a house, he lived in the forest, sleeping under trees with snakes and scorpions around. He advised me not to be afraid of them and just eat five leaves. I didn't heed that because I was a city boy. After a week, I got scared and ran away. My education was left incomplete. On and off, whenever life became complex, I would think of him and I would get answers automatically in my head; I don't know how.

So, I started treating people. This is my hobby—not a profession or business. I had to start manufacturing certain things myself, like Moringa oil, Tulsi water, Ajwain water, Bel patta water, because I could not depend on people to get the quality required. I started treating cancer patients too. Today, more than 100 cancer patients have survived very comfortably for over ten years. Dinesh Bhai Kotak, whose colon was cut by 18 inches in 2012, came to know about me. He didn't go in for chemo and radiation; he came straight to me. I treated him with Tulsi water and Bel patta water, and, today, he has reached the age of 91 years."

How does Naturopathy help cancer prevention and cure?

"There are various fields in naturopathy, but my work is with plants. I joke with people and say no matter which religion, all the Gods and Goddesses are kings. When they feel sick, they run to the trees; this is what our forefathers taught us, and we have been learning it for ages. So, I thought to myself that there was nothing better than nature. Whatever nature has given, you can be cured by nature itself. You have to go along with it to cure yourself."

What do you think are the major factors behind why people are getting cancer today?

"Chemicals are the main reason—spraying pesticides on food and fruits and reusing plastic for a long time brings you closer to cancer. Majority of things today are made of plastic. Even our food is packed in plastic bags, which we can't avoid today."

How to protect oneself from cancer?

"Try to live as naturally as possible. Go for good exercises. Wash your vegetables with soda bicarb and hot water and then in cold water to get rid of pesticides to the maximum."

If a cancer patient comes to you, how do you treat them?

"For cancer patients, I suggest around 1000 leaves of Tulsi per day. Tulsi contains the highest amount of antibiotics. And we offer it to over 33 million Gods and Goddesses. This Tulsi is the most powerful thing in the world. It also has chemo properties—1000 leaves per day is natural chemo suggested by me. I also wrote in Reader's Digest in the November 2014 issue that 1000 leaves a day for one month is natural chemotherapy with no side effects.

One cannot eat 1000 leaves a day. It contains a lot of mercury, so you can't chew Tulsi. I distil it so that mercury doesn't get into the water. Mercury is heavy, so it does not collect in the vapour that turns into water. The Tulsi water I give is mercury-free. Also, Bel patta is offered to Lord Shiva, known as all-powerful. His energy is in Bel patta. Once you consume both of these, within two to three weeks, say, a maximum of six weeks, you will say you are feeling better.

Stages of cancer are defined by doctors. As far as I'm concerned, it frightens the person into going in for chemotherapy, which causes a lot of damage to the body and helps the cancer spread everywhere. Cancer is the rotting of a fibre or fibroid to such an extent that it is known as cancer. And because you can't reach it physically, by giving it heat or radiation treatment, you end up spreading it everywhere in the body."

Most patients opt for conventional therapy because they are scared. Why do you think naturopathy or other alternative healing therapies are popular?

"The lobby of pharma companies is very powerful—it is ruling the world today. It is challenging to fight with them. They are a bunch—whereas a single person like me can't fight with them."

What about people who use chemo and radiation? Can they also opt for naturopathy?

"They can, but not together. Two chemos cannot go together because you will get blisters if you have Tulsi and chemo simultaneously and you won't be able to eat or drink anything. Even sipping water will be painful."

How long after chemo and radiation can you take naturopathy?

"After 20 days minimum, you can start."

How can one manage the side effects of chemotherapy?

"Carrots are good. You can cut some of the side effects of chemo with carrots and Tulsi, but not completely."

As per naturopathy, what are the early signs of systemic illness or poor health?

"When you feel so tired that you can't walk; you can't do your work. Wrong food habits lead you towards bad health."

If you have to point out five ways to prevent cancer?

"Two glasses of carrots a day is good enough. Tulsi juice of 100 leaves."

Can people with a history of cancer do something about it?

"They can avoid cancer by having carrots and Tulsi. Genes do play a part to a certain extent.

But it is better that one does not think about genes as the mind also plays a role."

What other illnesses can be cured through naturopathy?

"I have treated people with muscular dystrophy and achieved good results with Tulsi, Bel patta, and Moringa oil. Some diseases cannot be cured in any way, but these treatments can help to a certain level."

Any other suggestions for cancer patients? Is there any advice you would like to give them?

"You should not go in for chemotherapy — 65% of your intake should be carrots, and you should avoid milk and milk products. Sugar, when it is chemically processed, is harmful—so white sugar is out. Jaggery is much better. You don't have good honey because flower production is not there. And the amount of honey available in the market is all fake. Exercise and walking 1.5 hours a day will help cure cancer faster.

There is a tree bark from which powder is made. It removes all kinds of infections. For example, you can apply it on boils of any sort and the pain reduces within half an hour. For cancer patients, we recommend a three-finger pinch, which is about a quarter teaspoon. Boil. Boil it in half a cup of water and drink that. All the infections in the body or urinary tract, even UTIs, are cured with that.

And what about coconut oil? You use it to massage babies, for hair fall, pigmentation, skin itching and softening. We encourage cancer patients to drink one spoon of coconut oil so that the infected part is covered with that oil and the infection is thereby contained."

***

Dr Rashmi Menon. Leading Homeopath. *Dr. Rashmi Menon is a physician who heals without medication, helping patients reverse lifestyle diseases including diabetes and cancer.*

"I have been practicing since 1999 using classic homeopathy. Those days, the number of cancer patients was relatively less. I would help them deal with their ailments using constitutional homeopathic medicines. People were not very scared of cancer then and were open to holistic medicine.

Over time, cancer cases started increasing. What shifted also was the approach of the patients towards their disease. There came upon them a fear that was not there before, an impatience to start chemo and radiation, and a readiness to undergo surgery. All this was concerning.

Then came the cancer pandemic where every family seemed to have a cancer patient. What I experienced was that there was also a shift in the stage at which they presented. Mostly, they would come to me after they had exhausted all other avenues—when the allopathic doctors had told them to try experimental drugs, opt for palliative care, or given them a death date.

When patients come to me, their lifestyle habits need tweaking so that the body has the space to heal itself. When the body has already undergone surgery or is undergoing chemo/ radiation/hormonal/experimental drugs, it needs additional help. That help is provided through homeopathic medicines, naturopathic treatments, natural juices, and therapies. All these have to be customized to the individual; just as no two people are exactly the same, no two disease patterns are the same.

These days, the most critical job is to handle the terror that patients and their family members face when they hear the diagnosis. This takes intense counselling and psychotherapy. Even with personalized holistic treatment protocols, addressing the mind is the game changer that determines how fast and deep the healing can go."

A glimpse into how I started holistic practice:

"The five and a half years of medical college that I attended to attain a Bachelor's in Homeopathic Medicine and Surgery prepared me to see my patients as holistic personalities and not just a combination of body parts/systems. In homeopathy, much importance is given to the personality and mental makeup of the patient in order to choose the best treatment protocol for them. Importance is given to healing rather than looking for symptomatic relief.

As licensed homeopathic practitioners, we are trained not only in anatomy, physiology, forensics, pathology, prognosis, and diagnosis, but also to identify the nature, individuality, and psychology of patients to prescribe the best cure for them. Psychology piqued my interest, leading to post-graduate certification courses in psychotherapy and clinical hypnotherapy.

While the mind is being understood, the body cannot be neglected. Through my training in whole foods, plant-based nutrition, and advanced Ashtanga yoga principles, I combine them to see the beauty of healing without medication.

A journey that started in 1999 led to deeper understanding, unlearning, and learning, and it continues till today. I consider myself a student on this path every single day."

Three essential things a cancer patient should do after a diagnosis:

"First, understanding that like diabetes or blood pressure, cancer is a lifestyle disease where the body is trying to cope with faulty lifestyle habits. Pay attention to these three things:

1. Check what you are eating—eat whole-food, plant-based, chemical-free food with high-living food (uncooked food like salads) or raw food.
2. Practice stress-relieving exercises and connect with a counsellor. The mind

plays a significant role in how your body responds to treatment.

3. Do not neglect exercise. Do not overdo it either. If you can do your exercise amidst nature, it would be the best thing."

Why is changing your diet relevant?

"Food is the easiest thing one can change when it comes to lifestyle. We are what we eat. Each time we eat, we provide the raw material for our body to rebuild. The quality of the raw material will determine the quality of the body. If we eat highly processed junk food, the body gets hardly any nutrition. Instead, it is kept busy fighting the inflammation that these foods cause. Hence, food is the first thing one must look at when treating cancer and other lifestyle diseases."

My thoughts when Shruti first came to me:

"Given her young age, I thought her body had the capacity to heal itself, and getting off conventional allopathic treatment would help. However, the pressing goal was to recover from the side effects of chemo. Hence, I supported the allopathic treatment with juices and hypnotherapy, and used guided imagery just before a chemo session. A wholesome plant-based diet also helped her body recover from the assault of chemo."

Some major drawbacks of conventional treatment:

"Conventional allopathic treatment is good as emergency medicine. However, there is a lot of uncertainty when treating chronic long-term diseases where that stream of medicine does not understand the cause. In such cases, the remedy ends up causing more problems. The side effects can be debilitating. Many times, cancer patients perish from the side effects of chemo and radiation instead of the cancer. When their lifestyles remain toxic, treating the symptoms only leads to the toxicity showing up somewhere else in the same or another form.

That's why, when patients are relatively young with no other co-morbidities, I advise them not to go in for conventional treatment but actively pursue holistic care. However, if co-morbidities exist and allopathic treatment is already on, then my advice will vary from case to case."

A final message:

"We all know what is good for us but not all of us do what we know. Prevention is always better than cure. Look at your lifestyle and make modifications. Eat as wholesome and plant-based as you can, work on stress reduction, and connect with nature to slow down. If we don't slow down to take care of ourselves, the body will manifest disease to force us to stand still.

And if you end up with a diagnosis, whether it's diabetes, cancer, or autoimmune, understand that your body has the power to heal itself; you just need to get out of the way. Getting out of the way means not increasing the body's workload by giving it unhealthy, unnatural food, stressful thoughts, and stagnant movement."

Chapter 21
Expert Doctor Interviews and Case Studies

Dr Leroy Rebello - Functional Medicine Doctor. Founder of Biotex (A premium brand of supplements in India)

Please briefly explain your journey. Why did you become a doctor?

"I was sick and suffering from an autoimmune disease. I went to many doctors to seek treatment. I was given the normal course of therapy that included steroids and immunosuppressants; it only made me worse. That's when I decided to enter the field of functional and holistic medicine. After switching to holistic medicine, I healed myself and am doing very well now."

How did you receive this diagnosis? How did you understand it was an autoimmune condition?

"Many doctors diagnosed it—the best in the country and probably, the best in the world.

They did all the blood tests and said it was an autoimmune disorder and there was nothing that they could do about it. So, I had to start taking things into my own hands and treat myself.

I went on a plant-based, mindful lifestyle. I started a course of different meditation practices and exercises. When you go to a doctor, they tell you to try meditation. How does one meditate? What to meditate on? Nobody explains that. What exercise to do and how to exercise? What is the right equipment to use and how to use it? Should you go to the gym or not? So, I had to do a lot of research and find out for myself. Gradually, that's what helped me move ahead.

Before the diagnosis, I was practicing dermatology and cosmetology. Now, I've left that behind and I'm practicing completely conscious medicine. I wouldn't call it medicine, I call it a 'conscious life practice'. I help people change their lifestyles."

When you changed your lifestyle, did it resolve your condition?

"It's almost completely reversed, about 80-90%. I'm still working on the remaining 10% using Biotex. Biotex makes whole-food plant-based supplements. These supplements are 100% chemical-free. We go to the fields, chant certain mantras, and pray to the plants. We ask their permission to plant on certain days of the calendar year to get the right amount of active ingredients in them. And that's what we use for treating patients. Everyone who has experienced a Biotex supplement says they are happy and that it brought good changes in their lives."

We've been working with a lot of cancer patients who take your supplements. From the view point of functional medicine, what do you think cancer is?

"Basically, cancer is an overgrowth of misprogrammed cells. The misprogramming happens because of bad lifestyle choices and the epigenetic factors surrounding people. So, these epigenetic factors must be taken care of—people must change their lifestyles and live happy lives. There's also something called the 'micro-environment'—the environment that's within yourself. So, one needs to look within, find peace of mind, and meditate well. And if someone has cancer or the risk of cancer, that risk can come down. Studies show that even having the right diet, especially with a lot of coloured foods help.

Many of you know lifestyle changes will happen if one embraces a plant-based conscious lifestyle."

For a lot of people diagnosed with cancer, their first reaction is to start conventional therapies like chemo, radiation, and now, immunotherapy. What is your take on this?

"I wouldn't suggest not going to the doctor, but I will say go to a conscious doctor who understands all modalities of treatment because cancer is a complex disease. You should find a doctor to guide you who is into functional medicine—one who has good knowledge of cancer. And one who can also use some modalities of modern medicine to give you the best outcome. The cancer should be cured, and you should live a cancer-free life."

You are talking about an integrative oncologist, right? However, it's difficult to find a good integrative oncologist in India.

"Many oncologists have started using integration in their practice. I wouldn't say it's difficult— they say you can find God if you search. So, I think we have to just search for the right one."

There are a lot of myths about taking supplements during cancer treatment. What is your take on this?

"The supplements you take during cancer treatment have to be the right supplements. For example, during cancer, you lose a lot of weight and protein, so you need a lot of amino acids to build up your protein and not the once that contain glutamine which promotes the growth of cancer. So Biotex offers aminos without glutamine.

Most oncologists prescribe antioxidants; high doses of Vitamin C also work very well. Each person will have a different treatment protocol according to their sensitivities and needs."

Despite going into remission, many people have a relapse. How can we prevent a relapse?

"According to me, a relapse basically stems from the lifestyle followed. If you make the right lifestyle changes you can avoid a relapse. Maintaining emotional health is important too. You need the right prayer practice and support from family and friends. That always helps during tough times. Some people are lucky enough to have that, and for those who don't, it's essential that you search for people who can help."

What roles do genes play in developing cancer?

"There are specific genes that put one at a high risk of cancer. But these genes are impacted by epigenetics. So, it is not necessary that if you have the genes for cancer, you will get it. If your epigenetics are right, you will be fine."

***

Dr Sachin Gupta - Integrative Oncologist at Max Super Speciality Hospital, Mohali

Would you like to share your journey? How did you become interested in oncology? What inspired you to enter this field?

"Thank you, Shruti, for having me in this conversation. I am the Director of the Medical Oncology Department at Max Super Specialty Hospital in Mohali near Chandigarh, and I've been working here for more than 12 years. I started this department when this new hospital came up in 2011. Before that, I was associated with other prominent institutes like Medano Hospital in Artemis Hospital, Gurgaon, DMC Hospital in Ludhiana, and Rajiv Gandhi Cancer Hospital in Delhi where I did my oncology training.

While doing my MD Medicine at DMC Ludhiana, I worked in the oncology department, where I got to understand cancer treatments. This branch fascinated me more than others—there was some inner call that always answered 'oncology' when I asked myself what my interest was. Maybe this was my charted path in this lifetime. Simultaneously, I follow a spiritual organization and a famous book, *Autobiography of A Yogi*. My faith and belief system come from there. The book introduces you to the concept of God, the guru-disciple relationship, and the laws of miracles. It talks a lot about healing yourself and your inner journey for self-realization. This was going on side by side with my training in MBBS.

As I went deeper down this path, I read many other books like *Love, Medicine & Miracles* by Dr Bernie Siegel. He talks a lot about how there are things beyond the medicine we practice that affect our health and healing. That's how the journey started. I went deeper into this. I have learned past life regression therapy, Reiki, and Pranic Healing. I connected with Blossom Furtado, a hypnotherapist in Delhi. I took some sessions, learned hypnotherapy, and practiced on patients. I found that there are tools beyond allopathy that can help patients by identifying the root cause of the disease. There are things beyond the physical body that are in the mind.

As you know, our body has a chakra system—an energy system. Blockages in energy flow can lead to disease in those organs where this blockage is happening. Now, where the blockage is happening depends upon what kind of emotional turmoil or other issues one is undergoing, so that may be a root cause. There may be guilt in survival issues. Or, there may be greed, lack of love, or a feeling of injustice. We harbour so many emotions and emotional traumas inside us, and over time, these things keep accumulating, causing blockages, and then diseases start appearing in the physical body.

Modern medicine doesn't discuss the energy system, the astral body, or the causal body. We are focused mainly on the physical body. I wanted to combine this knowledge with my practice and work on the physical body along with mind and soul medicine. We started doing workshops with Blossom. Every two months, we held workshops where we invited cancer patients and their families. We did guided meditation and discussed the nature of the soul, the power of mind, the power of belief systems, the power of affirmations, and goal setting. Then, the meditations revolved around forgiveness because forgiveness is a potent tool for release. So, we started teaching and doing all these things along with the routine treatment patients got from us. And we did see some wonderful results. Many patients could work on themselves; they could either move on from their relationship issues or mend their relationship issues through love and forgiveness triggered by this knowledge.

We had mixed results: some successes and some so-called failures. As healers, we must acknowledge that everybody is on their soul journey and we can't interfere in anyone's karma. We may try to help with guidance, knowledge, and meditation, but each soul must decide for themselves. We keep guiding them to take charge of their lives using willpower with this knowledge and do some extra work on themselves beyond physical medicine."

It's amazing to hear that. How do your peers react to it? Do they believe in your approach? Or do they discard these integrative practices?

"I found in my journey over the last many years that the doctors in my field have been quite open to it. In India, people are deeply religious. A common faith and belief system comes from our traditions, and we have the concept of a higher power to whom we pray. We try to connect to it using the principles of yoga and meditation. We may not practice it daily but we are aware of it. The doctors in my field are quite open to it and realize its importance.

But, it's a different matter that we cannot practice it ourselves because 99% of the time is devoted to the physical body. Our patients are in so much pain due to their physical bodies. The pain, the handicaps, and the treatments are also so diverse and so difficult. Whether chemotherapy, radiation therapy, or surgery, our time and energies are diverted into looking after the physical body. It's up to the patients if they want to do this. There are a lot of centres now that have holistic programmes, counsellors and psychologists.

The Brahma Kumaris, The Art of Living, and many other spiritual organizations are associated with helping these patients in their spiritual journeys in addition to physical treatment."

What if somebody doesn't want to take chemo or radiation now that people are reading about integrative protocols. People want to know about nutrition and diet as well. What are your thoughts on this?

"In my frank opinion, it depends on the kind of cancer. It could be a very mild kind of cancer that grows very slowly, or a very aggressive cancer that grows very quickly. Modern medicine is quite effective and established and has much to do with helping the physical body. Let's take lymphomas—Hodgkin's lymphoma, non-Hodgkins lymphomas... These lymphomas are quite curable with chemotherapy. Now, suppose a patient with lymphoma comes and says, "I will just do meditation and will take care of my life and cure my cancer"—I am not a person who will encourage that. Because in the present age, we are ascending to the Upper Yoga with the kind of understanding and scientific developments. The majority of the population is not going to get cured with meditation or with diet. Cancer has already developed, so we have to use physical methods.

I always tell my patient to remember how Lakshman*ji* was injured and unconscious in the Ramayan, and then Hanuman*ji* had to bring the Sanjivini *booti*. Even when Bhagwan Ram was there by his side, he did not do energy medicine to heal him. He did not do *chamatkar* to heal him. He did not ask him to meditate or do yoga. Physical medicine was required at that time. Similarly, physical medicine is also created by the higher power of God. Even medicines come from chemicals or plants that have healing properties. So, we can't disregard physical medicine. It is a God-given power. Surgery, chemotherapy, and radiation are critical, and they help in curing lakhs of stage 1, 2 and 3 patients and prolong the life of stage 4 cancer patients. I won't recommend that anybody quit medical treatment and go in only for alternative methods. But integrative medicine aims to combine these things. Allopathy takes care of the physical body and helps cure the patient; alternative and energy medicine helps in that journey.

I mentioned that relationship issues could be the root cause of energy blockages, so we need to remove those blockages. Then the patient becomes more receptive to the treatment, and can apply this willpower to make lifestyle changes, and take care of diet and nutrition. Modern medicine lacks advice about diet and nutrition because we focus more on the treatment and medical protocols. Some practitioners suggest the wrong nutritional items to patients. They keep them only on, let's say, a liquid diet, or only on fruits, and the patient becomes weak. A cancer patient needs a lot of protein and energy. So, I encourage my patients to have a nutritious, plant-based diet with adequate proteins. They should also add fats, lots of fruits and vegetables, and salads and juices wherever they are not contra-indicated due to their condition. If somebody has some food preference, we leave it to them—for instance, if they want a non-vegetarian diet. But I generally advise them to go for a plant-based diet, adding adequate fruits and nuts to the treatment. Saying that you will heal your stage 2, 3, or 4 cancer simply with meditation or yoga or only nutritional changes, I don't believe it can happen.

We live in an era of modern medicine where many targeted and immunotherapy medicines are miraculous cures for some patients. Of course, they are not for everybody, not for all diseases of all the organs. Still, in certain diseases, allopathy has excellent medication to offer, even for stage 4 patients, and has the potential to cure stage 1, 2, and 3 patients."

I wanted to talk about supplements because there is a lot of confusion about them. Some doctors advise supplements while some doctors say they interfere with the chemotherapy or the radiation. What is your take on this?

"Generally, we don't give too many supplements during treatment, but patients are advised on a case-to-case basis. Some of our patients are nutritionally challenged—like somebody who has cancer mainly due to anorexia and loss of appetite. So, patients may have been eating poorly for many months and developed some deficiencies. These deficiencies may be in the form of a lack of calcium, magnesium, and other salts, especially iron. Vitamin D deficiency is rampant as most of us sit indoors and work. Vitamin B-12 deficiencies may be due to poor nutrition and poor absorption of nutrients from the gut, so we remedy that with suitable supplements. Overdosing on these vitamins does not aid healing. In some cases like vitamin B-complex, the extra vitamins get excreted in the urine, not accumulated in the body. Bombarding a patient with supplements is not going to cure cancer."

What about hydro-vitamins, CIVS, and ozone therapy? What is your take on these?

"Ozone therapy helps in certain areas. Again, it is part of an approach for patients. We don't claim to cure patients with ozone therapy and no other treatment. Better oxygenation and ozone decrease inflammation; in certain cases, it helps build tolerance and treat some infections. But sometimes, it can also increase the side effects. It is not a substitute for primary treatment."

We live in a pool of toxicity. Toxins are in the environment and food and are one of the leading causes of cancer. So, how does one remain cancer-free in this world?

"In this part of the world, farming practices have changed significantly in the last 60-70 years, and farming now has too many chemicals. Crops and seeds are genetically modified. And we are heavily dependent on fertilizers, insecticides, and pesticides. All this has come into our food, and, of course, is affecting us. Even milk-giving animals are given injections of oxytocin and other things to increase milk production. The greed for more production has led to all this.

When I became cognizant of the damage of chemicals, some inspiration came. We started an organic farming community six years back with about 50 member families where we grow our vegetables. We have a lot of fruit trees divided amongst us. We are promoting awareness so that more and more people start group farming, lease some land, grow their vegetables, and develop kitchen gardens. People should ask vendors for organic food and pressure society, governments, and farmers to go organic."

What about pollution? How do we deal with that?

"A lot of things have to come from self-discipline. And from putting pressure on governments and non-governments. Even though everybody is busy with routine work, whoever has this awareness must challenge everything that is happening. Laws are already there, and much work is being done, including by governments. We are moving to more renewable sources of energy. Vehicles are changing, and we are harnessing solar power and wind energy. These things will increase the use of renewable energy sources, and we will rely less and less on fossil fuels. Hence, the pollution situation is going to improve. But again, a lot of work needs to be done in this regard. Wherever we can contribute to decreasing carbon emissions and living a more organic way of life, we should do our bit—for example, by using a cycle if you have to go nearby rather than using your car, avoiding the use of too many gadgets and machines, and doing away with plastics as much as possible. People are coming up with innovative solutions, and things are improving. But you need laws, you need the execution of those laws, and you need penalties. And you need self-discipline."

Can you share a case study where you integrated both practices for one patient?

I remember a young girl who came to us with an ovarian tumour. She had a germ cell tumour of the ovaries and underwent surgery for the removal of those tumours, though her uterus and the other ovary were preserved. She was unmarried and had lost her father when she was only 4 or 5 years old. She was not from a very well-to-do family and had financial constraints. We were doing chemotherapy to cure the tumours. Now, this girl held a grudge against her father. So, I did a hypnotherapy session with her during her treatments at the hospital. During one of these sessions, she saw her father's soul as a bright light. We also facilitated a conversation with her and her father about her grudge. She asked why he left her when she needed him. As he was not there for her as a provider, she didn't have the kind of life she would have liked. She was harbouring this grudge and anger; all these feelings were there. Through the conversation she had with that bright light, she came to understand that it was a contract in this lifetime that her father had to leave early, and her mother had to learn to take care and increase her willpower and other faculties to live on her own and take care of her daughter.

Then she understood these spiritual contracts and that souls come and go. She understood that sometimes we must develop our faculties and powers, which is why these situations emerge. A lot of forgiveness happened in that session, and after that, she could move on in her life without grudges. Her tumour was cured. She got married, had a baby, and got a good job. It's many years now, and she sometimes comes just to meet me, and for a check-up. This is how spiritual understanding helps in life. I'm not saying that this would have cured her of cancer by itself, but it helped her.

I feel the manifestation of any disease in your body, starts in the emotional body. For many women who have ovarian cancer, I see a massive link to their dysfunctional relationship status. Many patients contract cancer within a few years of divorce and heartbreak. Their chakra system from the root to sacral is affected and off-balance. There is a direct correlation, though cancer is multi-factorial. It is not just relationship grief that causes cancer but physical factors as well."

What do you suggest for anybody who has just got diagnosed with cancer? What are three things they should do in their daily routine?

"Apart from conventional treatment, they should work on their inner self. They need to set an ideal place in their house where they can sit and pray, make an altar, and ask for help from the

Universe, according to their faith. Each of us knows there is a higher power in the Universe, a higher intelligence guiding us all the time. That intelligence has created all of us. So, we need to connect with that higher self and power and draw inspiration and energy from it. Sitting in meditation or silence gives us the answers to many things. We start questioning ourselves regarding 'Who am I?' 'Where have I come from?' 'What is the purpose of my life?' We wonder about our relationships and how things develop. We have an inner sense of knowing once we start confronting these questions which tells us the root cause of the problem. There is a sense of hurt, grief, or lack of love, which we keep inside. Self-love is absent often, and we are not compassionate to ourselves. Guilt is another feeling which is very damaging.

Being spiritual means smart living. This does not mean that you have to pray all the time, but that you are okay on the inside. Not being sad means spiritually living to your full potential and happily so that there is *ananth* state of joy and bliss. Once we identify the problems, we try to mend them with various tools.

Meditation is a tool, but it is not an end in itself. It is a means to an end. Meditation means listening to your soul, listening to the higher energies. It means drawing inspiration, willpower, and answers to your questions. Then, you work on yourself.

Another point is nutrition. We need to detoxify the body and eat lots of fresh fruits and vegetables with good chemicals that increase our immunity. Hydration is another vital thing alongside oxygenation, deep breathing, and do pranayama. Another thing is surrender.

For example, a new-born human baby is the most helpless creature in the world. If the mother doesn't look after her, it can't survive. So, if a mother cares for a helpless child, the Divine Mother can care for us when we are in a helpless condition. I always give my patients this analogy: 'You must surrender according to your belief system, be it to Jesus, Krishna, Divine Mother, or Lord Buddha.' These higher energies are there to help and guide us but a lack of faith holds us back. Lack of faith makes you question many things, and then you don't have confidence.

You need to have faith in your doctor and in the medicine you are taking.

Another thing, I tell my patients when their chemotherapy is on is, 'This is not chemotherapy. This is *amrit* going into your body. This is heavenly nectar healing your body, so don't take it to be chemotherapy because when you say chemotherapy, you are repulsed that something toxic is going into your body.' If you don't accept the treatment and if you don't have faith in the treatment, it is going to give you side effects. You have to prepare and channel your mind before taking chemotherapy—that it's going to help you rather than create side effects. That's so important because the cells start working that way."

What about insulin resistance in cancer patients? What are your views about sugar feeding cancer cells?

"Processed sugars are high in calories, carbohydrates, and even fats. I always discourage my patients from having too much sugary and processed foods. They can have a bit because we don't want to make their lives miserable and boring without some sweetness. So, a little bit here and there is okay. However, we should avoid processed sugars and replace them with natural sugars. We have fruits, honey, whole raisins, and dates that also give you a lot of minerals. One should avoid white sugar as much as possible."

What about dairy?

"Dairy is a very controversial topic. No species takes the milk of other species; only humans take milk throughout their lives. Many people have lactose intolerance and can't digest milk. I have understood that milk is not pure anymore because animals are not given proper diets and are given a lot of injections. We need to be very careful when choosing the source of milk if we consume it. Those animals should be fed well with a proper organic diet, and no injections should be given to them.

All the contents of milk are in nuts, so we can replace milk with nuts wherever possible. Almonds would have what is in the milk, so we can substitute regular milk with almond milk.

Human beings were designed to eat fruits and nuts. Our teeth, gut, digestive system, liver, and pancreas are designed to eat fruits and nuts. We have adapted our food and changed it so that we can eat many things. We are not intended to eat meat as we don't have long canines to tear the flesh, and our stomachs are not designed to digest flesh. But again, we adapted our food by processing, heating, and cooking so we can eat it."

***

I would like to mention here, Dr Sujit Chatterjee, founding member of The Other Song clinic, a homeopath and a cancer specialist. He supported my decision to forgo radiation and encouraged me to speak up and healed my suppressed emotions. Unfortunately, he's no more but I am so grateful to him.

Case Summaries

Many cancer patients have benefited from an integrative approach, the diet and lifestyle modifications and mental and emotional support offered by Awaana. I am presenting some case summaries and testimonials to demonstrate how integrative methods work.

Mrs. Kirti Lalwani's experience:

Diagnosed with ovarian cancer in February 2020, Mrs. Kirti Lalwani underwent surgery and recovered normally. Unfortunately, cancer was detected again in early 2021. She then turned to Awaana since she was resistant to the idea of undergoing another surgery and another cycle of painful procedures. She was suffering from disturbed sleep, aching joints and muscles (indicated by her high levels of ESR - inflammatory markers), and frequent headaches due to improper sleep, constipation, and poor energy levels. She had other complications as well, including hyperthyroidism, a history of gallbladder stones that were surgically removed, and she had undergone surgery for a hip fracture. Though Mrs. Kirti had a genetic background having seen both her parents go through cancer, she had faith in making a recovery and fighting the disease using natural and integrated therapies.

In the second phase of cancer, her energy levels were extremely low, and the thoughts of going through the treatment procedures were giving her anxiety and terrible mood swings. When she approached Awaana, she wasn't aware of what lifestyle changes she should make to manage her condition. Instead, she continued with the same diet and lifestyle. Our team recommended necessary lifestyle changes along with a diet programme to improve her low haemoglobin levels, reduce the toxic load of medicines, and support her recovery with positive results. She also wanted mental health support to overcome the emotional turbulence she was undergoing.

Nutritional approach

Mrs. Kirti's haemoglobin levels were low causing lower energy, aches, and pains. The side effects of various procedures contributed to weakness and weight gain. She was under multiple maintenance therapies, and post her IV therapy, her thyroid levels fluctuated even more. To combat that, a diet rich in phytonutrients and antioxidants was recommended to reduce oxidative stress. A stepwise diet plan was recommended to eliminate the side effects of chemotherapy, reduce inflammation (ESR) levels, and prevent a relapse by reducing certain food groups that make cancer cells grow faster.

Along with various detoxes, customized for her condition, a combination of anti-estrogen and anti-inflammatory diet was strictly followed. All animal-based foods were avoided (animal foods are carcinogenic in nature and trigger cancer cell growth). Herbs and supplements to reduce inflammation, like ashwagandha, Vitamin C, and certain fruits and vegetables, were added, and gluten was avoided to control inflammation. Switching to organic produce contributed to a reduced load of toxins in the body. Specific oils and spices were added to the nutrition programme to promote the healing of tissues.

Our integrative doctor, Dr. Milli, diagnosed her as being prone to cardiac toxicity and bone marrow depression due to a second round of chemotherapy with cancer relapse. To reduce these complications and side effects, she was given intensive therapies like high doses of Vitamin C, IV therapy, herbal pills, melatonin, and other nutritional supplements. This combination along with a micro-nutrient-rich diet that was completely plant-based helped to reduce weakness and mood swings and improved haemoglobin and B12 levels midway. She was also encouraged to practice yoga and relaxation techniques, which reduced oxidative damage to cells. She had put on weight with poor lifestyle habits and was willing to undergo recommended changes to bring all her symptoms to normal.

During her chemotherapy sessions, a support programme was introduced to reduce side effects that included certain high-antioxidant ingredients in the form of juices, coconut water, and detox drinks. The products she consumed in her daily life were identified and she was asked to switch from artificial to natural products to reduce the impact of false estrogens that come with chemical-based skincare and home products.

On May 22, Mrs. Kirti was given a prescription to prevent a relapse of the cancer by her oncologist. Due to the prescribed medication, she started having symptoms like headaches, weakness, and anxiety. She was then given an alkaline diet plan aimed at improving her low haemoglobin levels and reducing the side effects of medication.

This chart shows the comparative index of the symptoms the client faced before and after Awaana's Nutrition programme for 1 year 2 months: Ratings between 1-10 (10 being the worst and 1 being the least).

Severity of symptoms faced before	**Changes after the programme**
Acidity - 8	Acidity – 5
Constipation - 9	Constipation – 2

Headache – 5	Headache - 5
Pain – 7	Pain – 4
Disturbed sleep – 9	Disturbed sleep – 7
Skin dryness – 7	Skin dryness - 4
Energy levels – 7	Energy – 4
Mood swings – 9	Mood swings – 6

Changes in laboratory investigations/ parameters:

Test name	Recent values with date	Previous value with date	Reference range
Haemoglobin	9.5 (24-Sept-21)	10 (09-12-22)	12-15
Monocytes	7.6 (24-Sept-21)	0.21 (09-12-22)	0.2-1.0
CA 125	15.3 (24-Sept-21)	10.8 (09-12-2022	0-35
ESR	24 (4-Apr-22)	21 (09-12-2)	0-20
Peripheral blood smear	Microcytic hypochromic cells (anaemia)		
RBC Count	4.27 million/ m3 (24-Sept-21)	4.93 (09-12-21)	3.8-4.8/ mm3
Neutrophils	1.95 (24-Sept-21)	4.16 (09-12-21)	2.0-7.0

In Mrs. Lalwani's own words:

"My cancer was detected in 2020, and my surgery was completed in June. I was in recovery when I relapsed in 2021, and my chemo started again on March 2. I was very disturbed by this. At that time, my cousin told me about Shruti and Awaana Health and urged me to follow her diet. My daughter consulted Shruti and sent her all my reports. After reviewing them, Shruti recommended a diet plan, which my daughter helped me follow. I took this guidance while the chemo was ongoing and started seeing positive and encouraging results. Shruti spoke to me regularly and helped me a lot, giving me courage and helping me make my heart strong to face cancer. I felt the change happening within me. I stopped feeling weak and exhausted after the chemo.

Shruti was always available to clarify my concerns and advise me on the diet and lifestyle changes I needed to bring into my life. After the chemo, I would return to Jaipur from Gurugram the same day, and I used to feel good. The doctors wanted to give me medicine after the chemo but Shruti instructed me not to take the same, and I would feel good on most days. I was able to restart all my household work, and I felt quite normal. When I did another PET scan, the doctors said I did not need to have surgery again.

Following the diet, eating organic food and vegetables, practicing yoga, and meditation helped me immensely, along with the excellent doctors who cared for me. This was not my experience the first time I got cancer. After the first round, I became very careless and only realized later how big a role diet plays in cancer prevention.

Thank you, Shruti and the Awaana team who stood by me during my cancer treatment, responding whenever my daughter called and asked for guidance, even late at night. With the blessings of Guruji, I am now healthy and well, and no one can tell that I ever had cancer."

***

Nivedita Saxena's experience

- Conditions/Symptoms: Ca Breast pr+Her2 triple + ER positive, Hypothyroidism

Nivedita Saxena joined our Awaana programme in July 2022, taking up the Cancer 365 plan, where we supported her with nutrition advice, mental health guidance, and movement therapy for six months. At the time of joining, she was suffering from symptoms like weight gain, hair fall, poor sleep pattern, general weakness, frequent stomach upsets and occasional constipation, anxiety, and dullness of mood. Nivedita had symptoms like low haemoglobin that led to low energy levels, so we gave her an iron-rich diet and supplements that enhanced iron absorption.

This chart shows the comparative index of the symptoms the client faced before and after Awaana's reform programme for three months:

Symptoms/Issues faced before 25-7-22	**Changes after the programme 7-3-2023**
Pain rating on a scale – 8	Pain rating on a scale – 4
Hopeless about life	Feels positive and hopeful
Disturbed sleep	Can sleep without interruption

Changes in laboratory investigations/ parameters:

Test name	4/6/2023	16/1/2023	Reference range
RDW	13.5	15.9	11.6-14.0 %
Hs-CRP	3.7	6.5	<1.0 mg/L
SGOT	27	56	<35 U/L
SGPT	10	38	<35 U/L

In Nivedita's own words:

How did cancer change your life?

"Initially, when I was diagnosed, I went into a problem-solving mode. I was looking for a nutritionist and had one before I started working with Shruti. I was not convinced I was getting all the information. Shruti introduced me to various aspects of how I was supposed to take care of nutrition and suggested that I also look into spirituality. These things started helping me see things from a different angle.

For example, when going for chemotherapy, I always had a severe stomach upset, so I could not eat anything, even what was recommended. I could hardly keep anything down, so I only ate rice and *lauki ki sabzi*. But the moment I recovered, I tried following Shruti's recommendations. That helped me to bounce back faster after my chemotherapy was over. Finally, when I was done after six cycles of chemo, people used to tell me I was doing well because patients were often bedridden at this stage. I could take care of myself by following the nutrition recommendations, which helped my confidence."

How did it work for me?

"When I used to have acute acid reflux, I would immediately post a question in the Awaana WhatsApp group, asking what I could do about it. Almost immediately, someone would respond with a suggestion. They would tell me what to eat for instant energy if I couldn't eat anything for 2-3 days. These inputs may seem very small, but they helped me immensely.

Also, on Awaana's recommendation I did a few sessions on the spiritual angle. It took just one or two sessions to plant the seed that made me realize that I need to think about this aspect of my life properly."

What advice will you give someone who's going through cancer?

"When you get a cancer diagnosis, your first reaction is shock. Naturally, you will be very fearful for your life and the upcoming treatment. One thing I now believe in one hundred percent (based on my own experience) is that if you have a strong will to live and a strong desire in your heart to go on in this world and live your life, you can. People have different reasons for wanting to live; some want to live for their children, somc want to achieve something in life, and others could have other reasons. In my case, I don't have children, but I was very determined to live. I wanted to live for myself and I was very sure of that.

Cancer happened, but I was sure it had come to teach me certain lessons, which led me to have that desire to live on and change my life. My advice would be to keep that will to live strong. You can manage everything else, but if your will weakens then nothing will help. It will get shaky when things get tough, but you must cast aside those feelings and return to the desire to live. You can explore resources that help you, such as journaling, meditation with spiritual teachers, or even therapy.

Focus on nutrition and gather resources from everywhere. Don't meet people who put more fear into you. Make sure you are surrounded by people who fill you with positivity while caring for you. I didn't even watch movies that could trigger any negative emotions. While staying positive, allow yourself to be vulnerable on bad days, but always try to bring back your desire to live.

Never hesitate to ask for help and get as much support as needed. If you want people to do certain things for you, ask them. If you want people to pray for you, ask them. Because these are the things I did. I had a specific WhatsApp group of my friends, and I was clear that they had to go with me when I was going for chemotherapy or if there was any emergency. And I asked them to pray for me too. So, I utilized all the resources available in the world that I thought would help me. Cancer first happens in your mind and then manifests in your body. So, you must first heal in your mind, and the disease will be healed in your body. Take care of your emotions and mental health; your physical body will follow."

***

Reema Dhawan's case:

In March 2023, Reema was diagnosed with high-grade serous carcinoma of the ovaries. She had undergone six cycles of chemotherapy (Paclitaxel+Carboplatin), the last being on August 2, 2023. After the fifth chemo cycle, her WBC count was not coming up. Liver and bone metastasis was detected along with post chemo Tuberculosis (TB): Treatment for TB with anti-tuberculosis drugs (ATT) started on July 1, 2023. She also had a blood clot in the leg, in the iliofemoral area and was taking a blood thinner called Apixaban.

Health issues and challenges at the time of joining Awaana

There was some genetic predisposition. Reema's paternal uncle had abdominal cancer at the age of 60. Reena also had a history of seizures, for which she was on a prescribed course of Tegretol. She also had probable exposure to heavy metals from multiple dental fillings and root canal treatments. She experienced personal trauma due to the death of her father.

How we (Awaana) diagnosed the root cause, and made the client run tests to analyse the conditions and decide on our approach

Reema's first dietary changes showed a significant intake of potentially inflammatory foods. Her medical history indicated possibilities of drug-drug interactions affecting hepatic clearance. It also pointed towards possible heavy metal toxicity due to multiple dental treatments.

We identified nutritional deficiencies as well.

Our priorities were to:

1. Neutralize the side-effects of chemotherapy
2. Support recovery after surgery was planned on finding liver and bone metastasis
3. After recovery, upregulate detoxification of Connective Tissue Diseases and heavy metals

Reema came through post-chemo and post-surgery wonderfully well, but her blood parameters remained a challenge. The WBC was still not increasing. We knew we had to intervene with our cleanses. We started working on her gut to ensure elimination was not obstructed and supported detoxification with our liver and lymph cleanses. Once the toxins were cleared, WBC levels started rising.

- Her haemoglobin was low as were her energy levels so we recommended an iron-rich diet along with supplements to enhance absorption of iron.
- We monitored her progress and modified our approach when required. Eating out lowered Reema's appetite, so we suspected a mild intolerance to a particular food group. We started Reema on ginger shots before meals and her appetite came back to normal.

This chart shows the comparative index of the symptoms the client faced before and after Awaana's programme for six months:

Symptoms/Issues faced before April 2023	**Changes after the programme - Oct 2023**
Pain rating on a scale – 8	Pain rating on a scale – 4
Hopeless about life	Feels positive and hopeful
Disturbed sleep	Can sleep without interruption

Parameters	**Results**			
Dates	**18-1-2024**	**16-2-2024**	**Normal Range**	**Units**
WBC Count	3.06	5.79	4-10	thou/ microL
RDW	17.6	15.8	11.6-14	%
Absolute Neutrophil count	1.35	4.7	2-7	thou/ microL

In Reema's own words:

"I found there was a great improvement in my condition and symptoms. Immediate impact was visible on many parameters like bloating, energy levels, various blood markers, etc.

Apart from physical parameters, the Awaana team played an important role in keeping my motivation and spirits high. Whenever you speak to the team, you walk out with a lot of positivity and a stronger mindset which is imperative to fight cancer. The team is really skilled on all parameters—diet, physical health, mental health and above all highly patient, empathetic and always available for you. Their personalised plans make a clear difference.

I look forward to continuing my journey with the team."

***

Smriti Suval's experience:

Smriti Suval was diagnosed with a rare metastatic cancer in the kidney. At Awaana, we checked her reports and, more importantly, understood her symptoms and tracked her eating habits and lifestyle. We found that she was genetically predisposed to nephrotic cell carcinoma because of the SBHD gene mutation. Her diet included potent cancer-promoting foods, and despite being aware of the triggers, she was unable to consistently enforce lifestyle changes and often fell back into old patterns.

We worked with her pre and post-surgery on dietary patterns, immunity, and regaining strength. However, after recovering post-surgery, there was a discontinuation. Smriti joined us again in 2023 following a relapse. She had been prescribed immunotherapy with Nivolumab and Ipilimumab. We were well aware of her suboptimal gut health, a long-standing obstacle in her case. We, therefore, started aggressively repairing and building back her gut instead of just supporting her to counter the ill effects of conventional medicines. We started her on probiotics, supplemented with gut-repairing superfoods. We also introduced energy psychology sessions to heal her inner child, which was unheard of before.

Her mental health status:

Please complete the following sentences	8th Feb 2022	22.12.23
I am	useless	hopeful
If I die today	people around me will be happy	I tried my best
I have achieved	nothing	peace with what is happening

My life is	kat rahi hai	roller coaster, and I am enjoying it
I pursue these activities for pleasure	listening to music	watch TV, go for walks, cooking

Smriti's immediate goal was to prepare her body for surgery and post-operative recovery and prevent a relapse in the long run. We started her on a diet plan to prepare her for the surgery as well as to decelerate her metastasis. Post-surgery, we started yoga to regain strength and worked on emotional health, an aspect that had been overlooked so far. Low HB led to low energy levels, so we prescribed an iron-rich diet and supplements that enhanced iron absorption. We shifted her from animal proteins completely to plant proteins. We also stopped dairy products that were causing stomach irritation and reflux. The GERD symptoms gradually subsided once we put her on easily absorbable plant proteins.

The chart below shows the comparative index of the symptoms the client faced before and after Awaana's ***Integrative Cancer Therapy Programme*** *for three months:*

Symptoms/Issues faced before 2023	Changes after the programme 2024
Pain rating on a scale – 8	Pain rating on a scale – 4
Hopeless about life	Feels positive and hopeful
Disturbed sleep	Can sleep without interruption

Liver Function Tests	Current Levels (5.3.2024)	Normal Range	Units
Albumin	4	3.9-4.9	g/dL
Globulin	3.2	1.5-4.5	g/dL
Bilirubin (Total)	0.4	0.0-1.2	mg/dL
Alkaline Phosphatase	58	44-121	IU/L
SGOT	17	0-40	IU/L
SGPT	12	0-32	IU/L

***

Anitha Balaji's experience with Awaana

Anitha Balaji, a 47-year-old resident of Chennai, was diagnosed with Non-Hodgkin's Follicular Lymphoma in August 2022. Battling IBS, thyroid issues, anxiety, and fatigue, Anitha was on the verge of starting chemotherapy when we began optimizing her diet with rich phytonutrients and ensuring adequate levels of Vitamin D and B12. We recommended natural boosts like wheatgrass juice and Giloy to support her white blood cell counts.

Despite contracting COVID, Anitha managed it without complications, thanks to these interventions. We also encouraged meditation and yoga to help her manage stress and alleviate anxiety. After six chemotherapy sessions, her scans cleared, although she experienced side effects such as tingling in her hands and feet and persistent fatigue. To address these, we focused on building her immune system through juices and probiotics, supplemented with Vitamin C and curcumin. By January 2023, Anitha returned to work after regaining her strength and overcoming fatigue and anxiety.

How did cancer change your life?

"I realized I was not invincible. Life can take a turn anytime. We need a lot of close friends and relatives around us to support our journey. I understood that cancer is not a death sentence. It helped me build patience, perseverance, and resilience. I understood the meaning of living in the present moment."

How was it working with Awaana?

"Since Shruti is a cancer survivor, I could relate well to her. Her holistic approach to healing was beneficial. All chronic diseases should be dealt with holistically as your doctor may not have the time or knowledge of yoga, meditation, diet, etc."

What advice will you give someone who's going through cancer?

Accept the reality, trust your doctor, and do not Google things. Instead, focus on building patience and resilience as you go through treatment. Cultivate a sound support system around you. Take a holistic approach to healing. Stay positive."

Afterword

The reason I shared these case histories here is because I want to show evidence that an integrated and holistic approach works best for cancer. Many doctors don't believe in the healing powers of nutrition and mental wellbeing, The survival rate for all cancers is 67%, but now more and more young people are getting diagnosed, and that is a major concern.

There is no doubt that allopathic treatments have several side effects, and to manage those side. effects taking another pill is NOT the answer. I hope this book inspires cancer patients and their families to keep an open mind and not restrict themselves to following blindly whatever their doctors suggest. It breaks my heart sometimes to see people suffer so much when all they need to do is change their diet and incorporate certain holistic protocols into their treatment. Either they are not aware of it, or it is not approved of by their doctors despite having evidence to the contrary. Sometimes it's a matter of personal choice—people don't want to come out of their comfort zones and change the way they are living. **Please remember, cancer comes to shake you up and as a reminder that things need to change.**

Whenever I share my journey with people, they say they are sorry to hear that I had to suffer so much. I tell them, "Cancer is the best thing that happened to me as it has given me my soul purpose and a mission which is to help and inspire people." So embrace what you are going through as there is a deep meaning behind it; accept the change with open arms and you will be surprised. I feel honoured and happy that I am able to be there for cancer patients. If I can be a part of the their healing journey, it's like my mission is accomplished.

There are many roadblocks but I am trying to simplify holistic protocols and give people the best solutions. I am also coming up with an affordable course on cancer, accessible to people from all over the world, along with a recipe book that is cancer centric, meditation and yoga. My dream is to have a healing space where cancer patients can come and rejuvenate. Cancer doesn't discriminate; it hits the poor and the privileged alike, but the poor suffer more due to lack of resources. Hopefully, one day, I will have the opportunity to do something about it .

At Awaana, we see clients from all over the world and I have witnessed that the suffering is same, people are just as scared and apprehensive, and the quality of their lives are just as affected. Why not take care of ourselves and look into prevention instead of treatment or management of diseases? There are so many things I wish I knew earlier; I could have prevented many health issues.

Some of us feel doomed after listening to a cancer diagnosis. A support system where patients receive proper counselling before and after the cancer treatments is missing. At Awaana, we try to support the mental aspects as well, when we go through a client's case, Finally, I want to say—I've witnessed miracles. I have seen people with stage 4 cancer winning against it. So, take heart, anything is possible.

Photo Library

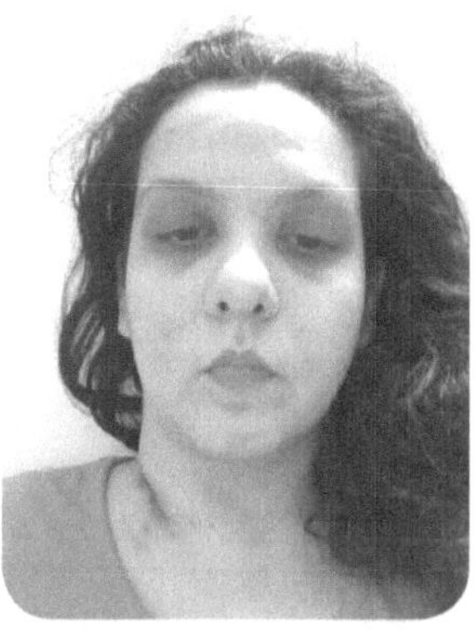

Hit by Cancer - Feeling Depressed and in Dillema, body is bloated and have no energy

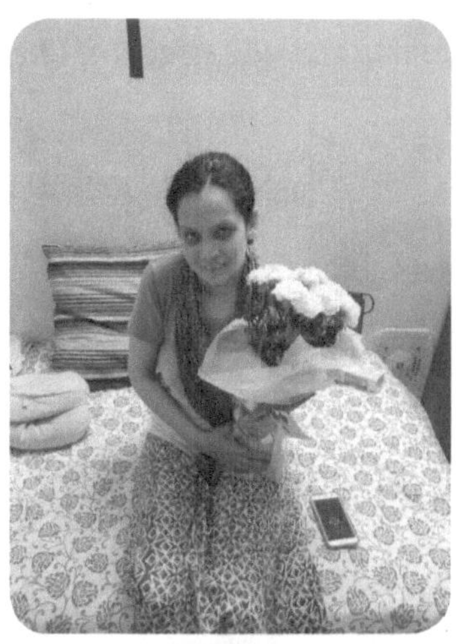

Trying Times - Started to loose weight & hair, still hopeful

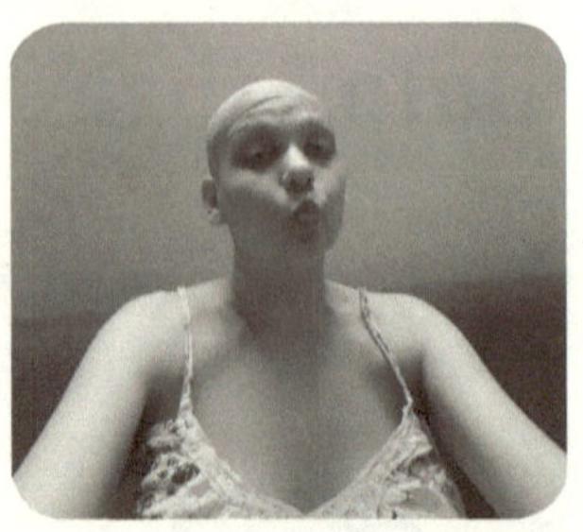

Embracing the new Look & Letting Go of any attachments

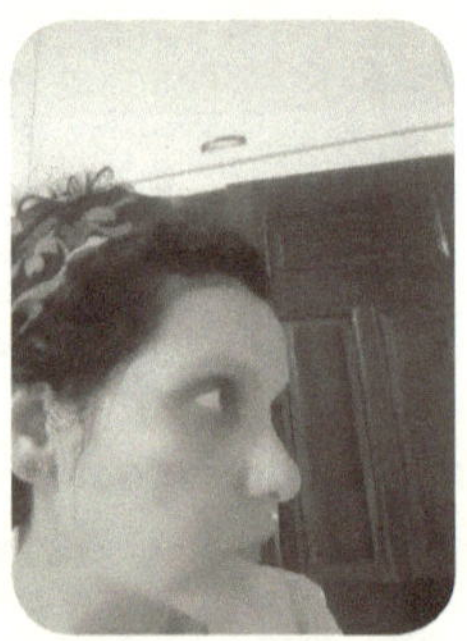

Detoxing the side effects of Chemo

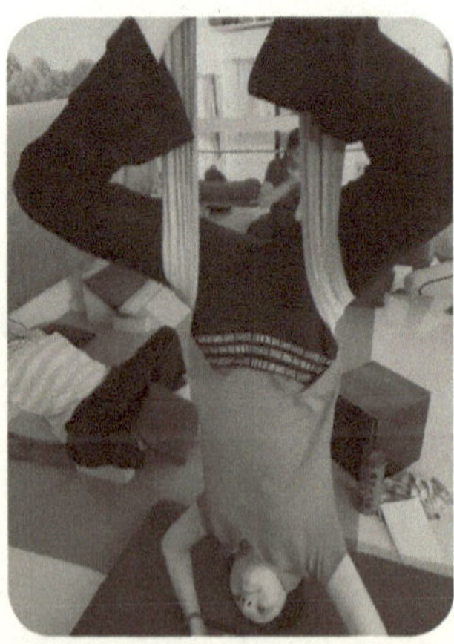

Building my immunity and strength with yoga and holistic therapies

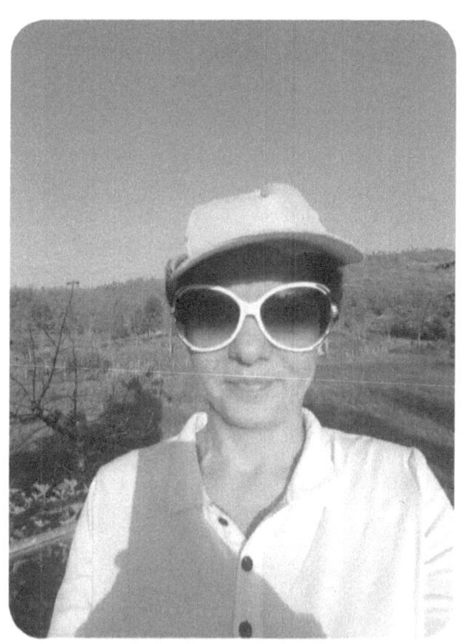

Enjoying sharing my journey & Motivating people by taking various workshops on Holistic Health

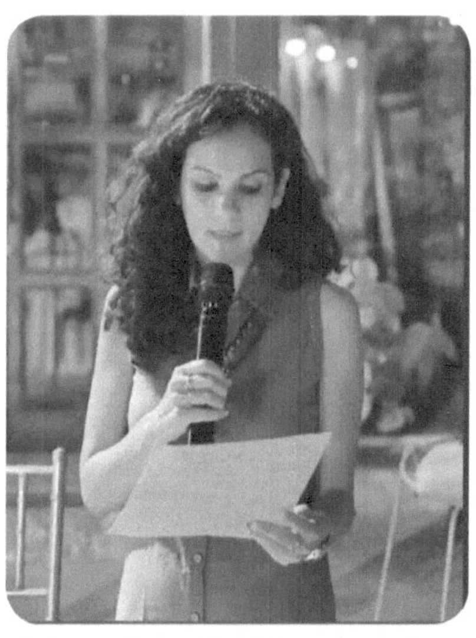

Started giving talks and taking workshops all over

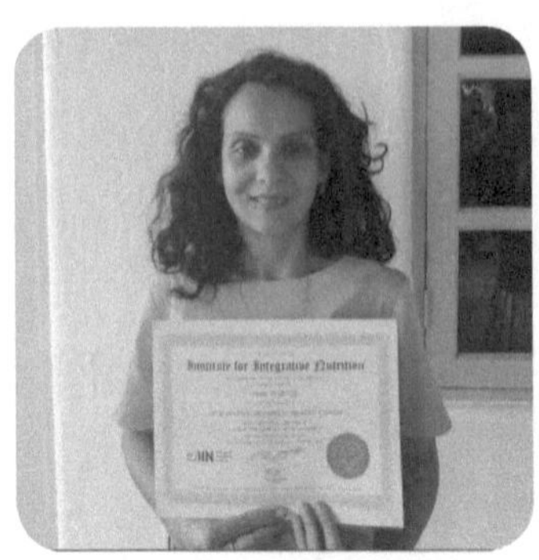

certified IIN health coach

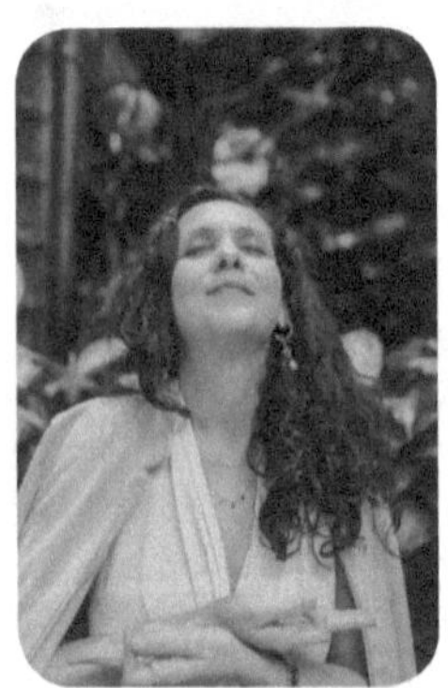

Shruti as Health Entrepreneur and Energy Psychologist

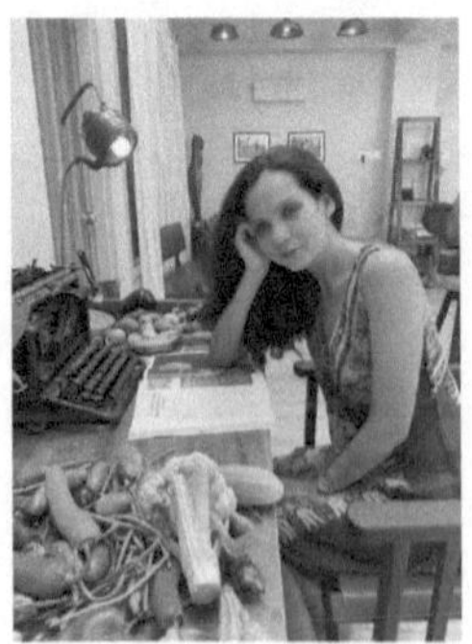

In the quest of learning more on Holistic Living

www.ingramcontent.com/pod-product-compliance
Lightning Source LLC
LaVergne TN
LVHW041206150826
845673LV00001B/304

9798892777964